5 ·10.09

Two in a million

Two in a million

A true story about illness and love

Ben Murnane

A. & A. Farmar

British Library Cataloguing in Publication Data
A CIP catalogue record for this book is available from the
British Library

ISBN: 978-1-906353-03-2

First published in 2008
by
A. & A. Farmar Ltd
78 Ranelagh Village, Dublin 6, Ireland
Tel +353-1-496 3625 Fax +353-1-497 0107
Email afarmar@iol.ie
Web www.aafarmar.ie

Typeset and designed by A. & A. Farmar
Cover designed by Kevin Gurry
Printed and bound by GraphyCems

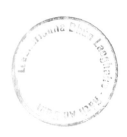

For 'Emma'
and for 'Aisling',
who made it possible

The house near Renvyle
(On writing my memoir)

I'm standing on the bridge
over our big stream,
or small river, the water

gushing in my ears, billowing
and stagnating around rocks
clustered in islands. Ash
from my last cigarette

falls in hot snowflakes
onto dew-kissed grass, smoke
caresses the rain . . .

I flick the brown butt into
the soaked bushes, and crunch
a path back to the cottage, my mind
heavy with words.

Shanaveagh,
Connemara,
September 2004

Contents

Preface   ix

Prologue: No excuse   1

1. The first nine years   3
2. No frills   12
3. Fartknocker   19
4. A boy and his steroid   23
5. Emma   29
6. Firsts   45
7. Expectations   61
8. Onstage   74
9. On the runway   91
10. Walk   102
11. Transition   104
12. Hell, part one   112
13. Hell, part two   127
14. Home   133
15. 'Now you turn around and tell me I'm not Jesus?!'   148
16. Tennis balls   163
17. A friend, a holiday, and some results   179
18. Maybe not forever   183

Epilogue: 'So'   201

Preface

Writing this book has been a humbling experience, because of the amount of help I've received. If I've left anyone off this list, I trust that I will be suitably chastised.

First and foremost, I'd like to thank my parents and my sisters. Mai and Des untiringly answered my questions, and Ruth and Jess, too, helped me recall memories that had become rusty. Mai kept a diary during my transplant. If I hadn't had access to the information in that diary, Chapters Twelve and Thirteen would not be nearly as detailed as they are. Des drove me around Dublin, from hospital to hospital, so my descriptions of the hospitals would be as accurate as possible. I couldn't ask for a more supportive family.

To all my friends, the ones mentioned in the book and not — thank you for your unending encouragement, and for your assistance when my memories of certain periods were incomplete. My thanks in particular to Michael Torrans, who is responsible for several of the descriptions in Chapter Three. I couldn't recall quite as much about Argentière as he could! Hugh Doherty is also deserving of special mention. He looked over the Epilogue for me.

I'd like to thank Terry O'Driscoll for giving me permission to reprint his 'Littal Buhrd' poem. My thanks to Kevin Hayes, for providing and for approving some of the info in Chapter Seven. Thanks also to Auntie Bing and Uncle Gerard, for consenting to my misuse of their identities.

My gratitude goes to Clare Sheridan, for helping with some of the info on BSP, and to Mr Godsil, for looking over a passage set in St Andrew's. Thanks also to Kristian Marken, for looking over some of the 2003 One-Act info. My thanks to Chrissie Poulter and Professor Brian Singleton at the TCD Drama Department, for checking some of the information in Chapter Sixteen.

My profound thanks to Dr Aengus O'Marcaigh, for poring over the medical information with me, for making calls and sending emails on my behalf — and for allowing me to misquote him throughout the

PREFACE

book! My thanks also to Dr Fin Breatnach, who tirelessly looked over drafts of some of the early chapters. Many thanks to Dr Gina MacDonnell, who helped reconstruct our therapy sessions, and to Dr Neil Adamson, for correcting some of my 'psychotic' mistakes. Thanks also to Dr Stephen Flint, for helping with some of the Dental Hospital info, and to Mary Ellen Eiler at the FA Research Fund, for correcting some of the details in Chapter Two.

My sincere thanks to the English teachers who helped edit this project—John Douglas and Mr Agnew. Mr A painstakingly unravelled my grammatical errors. JD spent hours trawling through my 'working' draft, making suggestions and pointing out what was crap. Bonus thanks go to John, whose idea it was to write the book in the first place. I'd also like to thank Eamon Grennan, who offered advice and support all along the way.

Thanks to the following people, each of whom helped with the 'post-writing' stage: Jonathan Williams, Eddie Rowley, and Cathy Soraghan.

Thanks to my publishers Anna and Tony Farmar, and to Katherine Farmar, my editor.

To 'Emma'—my undying thanks. I would not be me, without you. And this book could not exist, without you. Thanks for reading over everything, for supporting the project through everything, and for allowing me to turn you into a book character. Likewise, my thanks to 'Michelle'. The encouragement and the support and the suggestions—they've been overwhelming. Finally, to 'Aisling'—my friend and my hero. Thanks for giving me my ending.

Sources of medical information for this book include *Fanconi Anemia: A Handbook for Families and Their Physicians* Third Edition by Lynn and Dave Frohnmayer (Fanconi Anemia Research Fund, Inc., 2000) and *Fanconi Anemia: Standards for Clinical Care* Second Edition, edited by Joyce Owen, Lynn Frohnmayer, and Mary Ellen Eiler (Fanconi Anemia Research Fund, Inc., 2003). A lot of the descriptions of the symptoms of FA, etc. from the beginning of Chapter Two are essentially plagiarised from the Frohnmayers' Handbook—so thanks, guys, for that! Susan K. Stewart's *Bone Marrow Transplants: A Book of Basics for Patients* (Bone & Marrow Transplant Newsletter, 1992) has also been of use. Websites researched include vhi.ie (VHI Healthcare), ibts.ie (the Irish Blood Transfusion Service), bmdw.org (Bone Marrow Donors Worldwide), gaisce.ie (the President's Award), and rte.ie (Radio Telefís Éireann).

Readers should bear in mind that, while this book is a truthful account of my life as I remember it, dramatic licence has been taken with certain situations. For example, a conversation which took place via text messages may be written as having taken place over the phone; or, events from two hospital visits may be combined into one. Many conversations, particularly those with Dr Gina MacDonnell, have been condensed and/or improvised. Some descriptions borrow from articles I've written for *Totally Fushed*. It should also be noted that, while I was present at the Lindsay Tribunal on 27 February 2001, my memory of that day was not the best. Hence, some of the information regarding the day's testimony comes from news reports archived on RTÉ's website. All medical information in this book was believed to be correct at the time of printing. Any errors or inaccuracies are mine alone, and I apologise for them humbly.

This is a list of the people who have helped me specifically with the creation of *Two in a Million*. There are so many more people who have graced my life with their wisdom, insight, experience, encouragement, and assistance over the years that it is simply not possible to list them all here. Rest assured that you are far from forgotten. This story is (almost) as much yours as it is mine.

Prologue: No excuse

'You should write a book,' a friend once told me. 'Because serious illness is funny.' Hilarious, I thought. All those years in and out of hospital — the drugs, the blood transfusions, the catheters, the waiting lists, the pain . . . Just thinking about it has me in stitches.

I dismissed the idea. But my friend kept at it. 'Well,' he went on, 'maybe it's important that people like you tell their stories, to, y'know, offer hope to others.'

I snorted.

'Apart from anything else,' this ex-English teacher continued, 'I think it would be the kind of book people would buy. You could make money.'

Now I was interested.

I had been writing creatively since I was around seven years old, yet the thought of beginning a book was rather daunting. When I first spoke to another pal, also an occasional writer, about the possibility of penning a memoir, he joked, 'It must be nice to at least have a plot and characters worked out!' I smiled at that one. And if I had the plot and the characters, what excuse was there not to give it a go?

So, some months later, I started to organise memories into chapters, and began sketching the ideas that would eventually make up what you're reading now.

I hold no pretensions about this story — it's just one person's reflections. Some names have been changed (because I'm nice like that), though the essence of the tale remains unaltered. This is my life on paper.

But is it funny? You never know.

1. The first nine years

I don't remember much, of course, but this is what I've been told. My mother lay on the bed, hard in labour. The nurse was just putting on her latex gloves to help with the birth. Suddenly, I shot out from between Mum's legs and flew across the room. If the midwife hadn't caught me, well, it could all have been over before it had even begun! It was 3.01 p.m. on October the 23rd 1984, at the Rotunda Maternity Hospital, Dublin.

I was a small baby. Weighing in at just five pounds, I had to wear doll's clothes. My mum, Mai, would later tell me that, even at such an early stage, she knew there was something not quite right about me. I refused to drink from her breast, so her milk had to be expressed, and I was fed through a tube. My first few days were spent in an incubator.

However, it wasn't long before I was home, and began growing up. At the time, we lived in Loughlinstown, Co. Dublin, and my first educational experience was at a Montessori school in the area. I recall coming out of that school one day, holding my mother's hand. A young lad of three, I had a head covered in furious white curls. We passed a primly dressed lady who remarked on how cute I looked, exclaiming, 'Aw, the little angel.' I, however, was distracted by a larger boy some distance behind me, who was, for some reason, jeering at me. I promptly turned around and shouted at the bully, 'Ah, you're only a bollocks!' The taunting stopped. But no more nice comments were made — the lady hurried on.

Our family soon moved from Loughlinstown. We spent a year in rented accommodation in Mount Merrion, Dublin. While we were there, the crazy old woman who owned the house sent us notes scribbled on toilet paper every other week, asking us to leave. When we did finally leave Mount Merrion, we settled in the village of Kilmacanogue, near the town of Bray, in Co. Wicklow. I've lived in Kilmac ever since, in a house at the foothills of Sugarloaf Mountain.

I had a happy childhood. My parents were big fans of Connemara, Co. Galway, and my clearest recollections of those days before my diagnosis are not of Kilmac, but of Connemara — trudging up its granite-glazed peaks, frolicking with a rubber dinghy on its sandy strands . . .

The visits back to hospital started early, however. Before my fourth birthday, my parents took me to Our Lady's Hospital for Sick Children in Crumlin, Dublin, because they were concerned. Mentally, I was developing well (by the age of one and a half I could apparently hold full-on conversations with American tourists in restaurants). But physically, I was pale, and still slight for my age.

I went through a series of tests. The doctors did a bone scan, shoved a tube down into my stomach, and concluded that there was nothing wrong with me. My bone age was marginally lower than my chronological age, but this would correct itself with time, Mum and Dad were reassured. Nothing to worry about, nothing to see here, move along! For some unknown reason, though, nobody thought to take a blood test during that hospital session. I left Crumlin without consequence, and trundled along with my little life.

I went into Junior Infants at the normal age, attending the local school, Kilmacanogue National. I remember our class had great fun contemplating the wonders of the Magic Sweet Tin. The tin was magically sealed so that our teacher could only open it when we were good!

I went to Senior Infants at Kilmac National, as well. By First Class, however, I had moved to the multi-denominational Bray School Project. Our family did not practice any religion, and it had always been the intention of my parents to move me from Catholic Kilmac if I got a place in BSP, which was located just a short drive away. I was distressed at having to leave the school with which I was familiar, where I had formed friendships. But I would later look back on my years in BSP as some of the happiest I've lived through.

My first sister, Ruth, was born in 1988. In an attempt to prove just how obnoxious I could be, for the initial few months of Ruth's life, I perversely insisted on calling her 'Rory', making clear that I desired a brother in her stead.

Jess, my second sister, arrived just over a year after Ruth. I didn't have a problem with that name. My maternal grandmother, though, did. 'You can't call her Jess,' she told my parents, 'sure that's a dog's name.'

As the 1990s got into full swing, I was settling well into my new educational environment. I had made plenty of friends, with whom I enjoyed exciting playground games, including one where we pretended we were living in Candyland—a world of chocolate trees, minty grass, and candy floss clouds.

I went happily from First Class into Second. And from Second into Third . . .

And then they started. Sudden, excruciating, debilitating stomachaches. Mai thought I might have appendicitis, or something like that. But our family doctor couldn't see any underlying reason for the pains. As I started getting these aches, I also began to spot red dots on my skin. These would appear, last for a while, and then fade away.

Third Class went on, and I was feeling more and more tired, worn out. I didn't have as much energy as my classmates anymore.

But still, no one thought of taking a blood test.

One morning, my mum was listening to the radio, to a programme that was being broadcast from Our Lady's Hospital, Crumlin. There was a discussion on the symptoms of leukaemia. To my mother, some of the symptoms sounded very like mine—the paleness, the lack of energy . . .

Worried, Mai took me to our GP for a blood test.

I recall that morning, 24 November, 1993, the doctor taking my blood. I watched as he pulled the protective cover off the needle. The actual needle stuck out from a green plastic stem that had two wings; the wings looked like a butterfly's. The doctor gripped my wrist tightly, and then pushed the needle into a vein in the back of my hand. I felt a sting, and I saw red suddenly shoot up the clear tube that was attached to the green 'butterfly'. As the doctor observed my condition, he mused that I might have anaemia.

I remember chatting to a pal about the blood test once I got back to BSP. As we ambled around the playground during lunch break, I told him the fact that I had anaemia might mean that I would have to 'eat more meat'.

On the evening of Friday 26 November, the GP phoned with the results of the test. My mum picked up the receiver.

My blood counts were dangerously low. My haemoglobin (oxygen in the blood) level was less than half the norm—that's why my energy was zapped. I had ten times fewer platelets than I should. Because platelets were needed to aid blood clotting, every time I hurt or injured myself, I was at risk of suffering serious bleeding. My white cell count was virtually nonexistent. White blood cells were needed to fight infections.

'What are you saying?' my mum demanded.

The doctor said he couldn't rule out leukaemia. He recommended taking me to Crumlin Hospital immediately.

Mai hung up the phone. My dad, Des, returned home from work to find her in tears.

I had gone to a friend's house after school that afternoon. During the course of the day, I had developed a piercing pain in my ear — an infection. My friend's mum drove me home, and I complained about my earache to my parents once I got in the door.

Mai and Des told me that, because the pain was so bad, they were going to take me to hospital. There, I could get special medicine for the earache. My parents said that my granny, my dad's mum, would be coming to our house to look after my sisters while we were in the hospital.

I watched as my parents packed a bag of clothes and toiletries for me. And I remember feeling guilty. Mum and Dad had always told me to wear my woolly hat when I was in the playground at school. They said that if I didn't, I might get an infection. I never wore my hat — I thought it looked silly. Maybe that's why Mum and Dad now had to take me to hospital.

When we arrived at Our Lady's, the three of us sat in Outpatients for what must have been hours. I remember sitting on a bench along a corridor wall, swinging my legs back and forth to amuse myself, with the comforting buffers of my mother and father on either side of me. Eventually, I was given a bed in St Anne's Ward. I had a room of my own, with a television. The walls of my room were a calming sky blue.

The colour of the walls, however, could not calm my parents. Mai and Des were frantic with worry. They were discovering new things about my condition all the time. They learned that my stomachaches had probably seemed so severe because of my dropping haemoglobin level. The red dots on my body were called 'petechiae', and were caused by bleeding under my skin due to a dearth of platelets.

After the nurses gave me some drugs and my earache cleared up, I wondered why I was still being kept in hospital. Mum and Dad told me that I just had to have a few more tests, to see if there was anything wrong with me besides the ear infection.

I was going to have a bone marrow aspiration. I didn't really know what that meant, except that a giant needle was going to be stuck into my hip, and some jelly taken out. They were also going to stick a needle into my spine. I would be asleep while all this happened.

I left my parents at the door of the theatre. Once I was inside, I was shifted from my trolley onto the operating table. A lot of people in blue clothes were bustling about me. Odd-looking nets covered their hair, and they had masks over their noses and mouths or hanging around their necks. They were all wearing plastic aprons, and the plastic rustled as they walked. The ceiling was dotted with round white lights, like many moons.

A doctor peered down at me. 'We're going to give you a cannula, Ben,' he said. 'Did they tell you down on the ward what this is? It's a special tube that I can use to give you the medicine that will put you to sleep.' In preparation for getting my first cannula I'd had 'numbing cream' put on my arm a while earlier. After my aspiration, the cannula would stay in my arm, and could be used for taking blood samples.

'Keep your arm steady, good boy,' the doctor said. I raised my head from my pillow to see a needle a lot bigger than the 'butterfly' go into my skin.

Pain hit me like a flying cabinet.

And then there was nothing.

'Ben? Ben?'

'Uhhh,' I said.

'You just fainted. It's alright.'

The cannula was now stuck inside my arm, with the visible part of it taped to my skin. A syringe was attached to my cannula, and anaesthetic liquid was pushed into me.

Time to sleep again. I was challenged to try and count to ten. I don't think I made it beyond six. The world swirled around me, and things became darker and darker. It was as if I were falling down some endless hole; the light above was growing farther and farther away as I fell.

When I awoke, I was on a trolley in the recovery room beside the operating theatre, with wires attached to monitors stuck to my chest. There was a mask over my face, and oxygen was dancing around my nostrils. As I blearily came to, I daydreamed that I was a pinball, being bashed around by forces beyond my control.

I was wheeled back down to St Anne's. I could feel lumps on my hip and back, where cotton wool had been taped over the wounds from the giant needle insertions. Shortly after I got into my hospital bed, a thudding pain hit my back and my hip. The nurses gave me some painkillers, and these helped a bit. But I was still woozy; I'd never felt like this before—like all the world was a dream.

After my bone marrow aspiration, two or three days passed. For my parents, the wait was unbearable. Finally, some seemingly good news arrived.

I didn't have leukaemia.

The medical staff speculated that my low blood counts and earache might simply be symptomatic of a virulent virus.

But they were speculating without knowing the results of all my tests.

One afternoon, while my dad was elsewhere, a consultant came to see my mum. He stood in the hallway outside my room, and began to explain to a shell-shocked mother that her son had a rare disease called 'aplastic anaemia', and that he might have only six months to live.

It was then that a nurse suggested that before the consultant go any further, he take my mother into a consultancy room and at least allow her to sit down. The doctor did so, all the while continuing to divulge details of my condition to my overwhelmed mum, and showing no more sensitivity—according to Mai—than if he were 'listing ingredients for a cake'.

On account of this new revelation about my health, I was transferred from St Anne's to the oncology ward—St John's. I did not, of course, have cancer. But I might have had to undergo a bone marrow transplant, and John's was where they dealt with those patients.

In St John's I was under the care of another consultant, Dr Fin Breatnach—a kind-sounding man with grey hair and a grey moustache. He took my parents into a consultancy room and elaborated on what the other consultant had told them about aplastic anaemia.

It was an uncommon condition that resulted in bone marrow failure, which would have to be remedied with a transplant. In the meantime, there were drugs and other treatments that could be tried.

Dr Breatnach recommended I undergo surgery to get a 'Hickman' or 'Broviac' catheter inserted. The Broviac would go in through my chest and connect to a vein in my neck. From it, blood could be drawn; and, through it, intravenous medication could be administered. It was sort of like a more permanent version of the cannula. Cannulae lasted days—Broviacs could last a lot longer. Dr Breatnach said that a Broviac would prove very useful for me. I'd need to have blood tests for the foreseeable future, and the catheter would prevent me from being repeatedly prodded with needles. The Broviac could also be used to give me any intravenous treatments for aplastic anaemia I might have to receive. In addition, a Broviac is an essential piece of equipment for anyone undergoing a bone marrow transplant.

As he gave them all this information about my illness and outlined what he thought should be done, Dr Breatnach tried to calm my parents. He told Mai and Des it was a relief, at least, that I didn't have the genetic form of the disease, Fanconi anaemia, which could be a lot worse than mere aplastic anaemia.

But this was cold comfort to my mother and father, struggling to come to terms with so many life-changing facts at once. By now, relatives were looking after my sisters almost constantly, so Mum and Dad could both spend more time in hospital with me. They didn't know if they were going to lose their son.

I had been moved into one of the 'isolation' rooms, in the High Dependency Unit of St John's Ward. My immune system was extremely weak, and the HDU was the place where I could best be protected from infection.

I had my Broviac put in, which meant my cannula could be taken out. I was glad I wasn't going to be poked with any more blood-test needles. But it did feel strange, having this tubing inside me. I could see and feel the catheter under the skin on my chest, running up past my collar bone and disappearing into my neck. It was like there was a long worm burrowing into my flesh. I was now part boy, part medical equipment. The white tube of the Broviac emerged from my skin just above my right nipple. It then split into three smaller tubes, which to me looked like extremely thin penises with green heads. The nurses called the Broviac 'Freddie'. 'Freddie wants a drink!' they'd say, whenever the catheter had to be flushed with saline/anticoagulant solution — to clean it and to prevent blood from clotting in it. I thought all this 'Freddie' nonsense was quite unnecessary. I wondered what they called it when blood samples were coming out of Freddie — 'Freddie wants to puke'?

Soon after I arrived in St John's, Dr Breatnach ordered a second bone marrow aspiration. I thus had my third surgical procedure in a pretty short space of time. Oddly, by now, I was beginning to enjoy the anaesthesia, the sensation of blissful helplessness as the drugs conveyed me out of consciousness. When I awoke this time, groggy though I was, I decided to have a little fun with the medical staff. I said to the nurse who was watching over me, 'My computer brain is not working! My computer brain is not working!' Presumably she thought I was engaged in some form of drug-induced rave. Little did she know I was perfectly lucid, and getting my nine-year-old's jollies at her expense.

Well, I had to find fun somewhere. There was not much of it to be had most of the time in Our Lady's, after the novelty of watching television stations we didn't have at home wore off.

I might have felt even more bored than I already felt, were it not for my classmates in BSP. Our teacher organised it so that everyone in my class sent in his or her own personal 'get well' card. The cards included such touching messages as 'To Ben — the coolest gay around' (I'm pretty sure my friend meant 'guy'), and 'Niall Quinn Out Of The World Cup' (several friends were big soccer buffs, and Niall Quinn was my favourite Irish player). My class even compiled a book of puzzles, jokes, and poems, many of which they had written themselves, and sent it to me. They called it *The Ben Christmas Fun Book*.

In return, I wrote the class a letter describing all the tests I'd had, and gave it to my dad to drop into BSP.

A few days after writing this letter, I received another massive package of missives from my class. One friend, Emma, wrote in hers, 'Dear Ben, your handwriting is still good even though it looked a bit messy' followed by a rather wobbly and unflattering imitation of said handwriting. I was weak and sick — I had let my standards of penmanship slip!

In total, I spent just over a fortnight enduring hospital food during the winter of 1993. I was released from Crumlin in time for Christmas, which my family and I spent at home.

Like most kids, I loved Christmas. I loved the tradition of putting up the tree, and adorning it with both commercial trinkets and decorations I or my sisters had made. I loved the presents, of course, and the crackers filled with cheesy jokes and little collectibles. My belief in Santa was somewhat shaken by a friend of mine, whose parents did not allow Father Christmas to come to their house, but at nine years of age I was still prepared to accept that tale of the magical man in red trousers. The only aspect of Christmas I tolerated rather than enjoyed was the dinner. I was a pasta fan — I didn't understand why we had to stuff ourselves with turkey, Brussels sprouts, and potatoes every year. But my mum was a rigid Christmas traditionalist, and, on 25 December 1993, our family had a traditional Christmas dinner. And even though I'd rather have eaten spaghetti, it was nice to know that some things about life in the Murnane household weren't going to change. Since November, we'd been through a lot of turbulence, and we knew there would be more to come.

When the new school term started in January 1994, I was still too ill to rejoin my classmates. In February, I returned to Crumlin Hospital to begin a course of treatment for aplastic anaemia. This offered, according to Dr Breatnach, a thirty-five per cent chance of my life being saved.

My parents thought they knew where they and I stood — this would be our last battle, so to speak. Either we'd beat a-plastic anaemia, or it would end my life.

But the real story hadn't even begun.

On the cold February morning on which we walked into John's Ward, Dr Breatnach took Mai and Des into a small conservatory at the top of the High Dependency Unit. Toys were strewn about the conservatory's blue floor, and in one corner lay a broken foosball table. Fin Breatnach informed my mum and dad that some test results had come back from the genetics lab.

Then he got straight to the point.

'I'm afraid,' he said, 'that Ben has Fanconi anaemia.'

2. No frills

As the discovery that I had Fanconi anaemia came crashing through the door, the treatment I was about to begin for aplastic anaemia went out the window. It was a stroke of extreme good fortune that those test results came back from the lab when they did. If I had started the drug-intensive programme intended to reverse the effects of aplastic anaemia, I would probably have been killed.

The news that my illness was genetic changed things utterly. Aplastic anaemia was a bone marrow and blood cell condition — and a serious one. But Fanconi anaemia affected so much more.

FA gets its name from Guido Fanconi, a Swiss paediatrician. In 1927, Dr Fanconi published the results of his observations on brothers who had inherited various physical abnormalities, and who all experienced bone marrow failure. These patients could not successfully combat infection. They were chronically fatigued. They lacked sufficient platelets, and because of this suffered spontaneous bleeding.

Research has shown that, if both parents have the same defect in one of several 'FA genes', there is a one in four chance that any of their children will inherit Fanconi anaemia. About two out of every million children are born with the disease.

FA patients can experience a plethora of birth defects. Abnormally short stature is one of the most common. Babies may be born with hand or arm problems — for example, misshapen or extra thumbs, or missing arm bones. Kidney problems, such as having only one, are also common. Many Fanconi patients suffer 'hyperpigmentation' or café-au-lait spots — patches of darker discoloration on the skin. Some FA babies are born mentally retarded, others have low birth weight and may be slow to develop. Many patients have heart problems, as well. Male patients sometimes have underdeveloped genitals; female patients can experience puberty late and menopause early.

It's quite a cocktail of symptoms. But almost all FA patients eventually suffer complete bone marrow failure. What happens is that the bone marrow begins to malfunction and, as a result, normal blood cell production declines. This leads to anaemia — when the body experiences a scarcity of oxygen-carrying red cells — resulting in weakness and perpetual tiredness.

With the drop-off in bone marrow activity, the body also grows low on white blood cells. This means FA sufferers are uncommonly vulnerable to common germs. Plus, as already suggested, the low platelet counts FA sufferers must deal with can lead to excessive bleeding or bruising from the smallest of knocks. A dearth of platelets can sometimes result in internal bleeding, which can be fatal.

I have been lucky in many ways. Apart from double-jointed thumbs, mild hyperpigmentation on some areas of my skin, and my below average height, I have been largely spared the physical abnormalities associated with FA. And I was not born mentally retarded.

Yet the implications of having this severe illness go beyond the way one is born, and beyond bone marrow failure. FA patients are hundreds of times — in some cases, thousands of times — more likely to develop cancer than members of the general population. Cancers of the head and neck are particularly common. Fertility is reduced in FA patients. Women with the disease often have difficulty becoming pregnant; and, as of a few years ago, only three men with FA were known to have fathered children. Even if a sufferer of Fanconi anaemia undergoes a successful bone marrow transplant, he or she will not be free of this illness.

The average life expectancy for a person with Fanconi anaemia is twenty-two years of age.

On that February morning in 1994, my parents sat in the conservatory of the St John's High Dependency Unit, trying to take in all the information about FA that Dr Breatnach was giving them.

They'd been prepared for a final battle with aplastic anaemia. They weren't prepared for this. It was hard not to wonder whether the entire rest of my life was going to be mapped out by my newly re-diagnosed disease.

Instead of admitting me to Our Lady's, after he had given my parents all the Fanconi-related information they could handle, Dr Breatnach sent my mother, my father, and me home that same February morning.

With the discovery that my illness was genetic, it was decided that my sisters should be checked for FA as well. A few days after that heartbreaking discussion in the HDU, Ruth and Jess were taken to Crumlin for blood tests. The results of these tests would not be known for about two weeks.

My dad remembers the day the results were due, a Friday. He and my mum had arranged to go to a movie that night — the comedy, *Mrs Doubtfire*. My sisters and I were to be looked after by a babysitter. Dad rang up the hospital from work to get the results.

When he got them, he didn't phone my mum straight away. He drove home that evening, and the two went to the film together.

After the movie, my parents were walking the chill, streetlight-lit Bray roads back to the car, when Des told Mai the test results.

Mum burst into tears. Then she started screaming.

Jess had the disease.

To find that one child had a life-threatening illness was a huge blow, my dad recalls. To discover that a second did as well was 'pretty devastating, really'.

In truth, my parents had long suspected that if I had some disorder, Jess would have it too. She had many of the same features as me — pale skin with café-au-lait patches, wonky thumbs . . .

Thankfully, to this day, Jess has never displayed any symptoms of bone marrow failure. As I write this, she's as healthy and as annoying as a little sister should be. And long may it stay that way! Well, the 'healthy' part, at least.

There was a sliver of good news amidst all the grief that Friday in February '94, as well. Ruth did not have Fanconi anaemia. Not only that, but her bone marrow was a match for Jess's.

This could make things a lot easier for Jess down the line. Over two-thirds of transplant-needing patients do not have matching donors in their families. In each of these cases, an unrelated donor has to be sought. The fact that Ruth was a match meant that Jess would be guaranteed a marrow donation.

Freshly extracted marrow is the most reliable and most useful for a transplant. But it is possible to use marrow that has been frozen and then thawed. Some months after it was confirmed that her sister had FA, Ruth went into Our Lady's to have a sample of her bone marrow extracted. This marrow is being kept on ice. Even if something unthinkable happens to Ruth, Jess will still have a good chance of surviving, when the time comes for her transplant.

The only possible 'cure' for the effects of bone marrow failure brought on by FA is a bone marrow transplant (BMT). As with blood donors, bone marrow donors have to be compatible with transplant recipients. Only with bone marrow, there are a lot more than four major groups.

Early in 1994, members of my immediate family were tested as possible donors for me. Neither my mum nor dad, nor either of my sisters, was a match.

Then members of my extended family were tested. But my good-for-nothing aunts and uncles showed up negative as well.

In Ireland, there are over sixteen thousand potential donors listed on the Unrelated Bone Marrow Registry. From blood these potential donors have given, their tissue types are known. These tissue types can be matched against the tissue types of transplant-needing patients. The Bone Marrow Donors Worldwide database boasts access to over ten million potential donors. In 1994, it might have been possible to find a matching unrelated donor for me either in Ireland or elsewhere. However, the statistical success of 'matched unrelated donor' BMTs was not very high back then. But new technologies and medical breakthroughs were driving success rates up constantly. So, the team in Crumlin felt the best course would be to hold off sending me to transplant until it was an unavoidable necessity.

In the meantime, Dr Breatnach put me on an anabolic steroid called oxymethalone, which would, hopefully, boost my blood counts and relieve the chronic fatigue brought on by FA.

But my being on oxymethalone did not mean that things could return to the way they'd been before my diagnosis. Far from it. I couldn't even go back to school. The risk of developing an infection that might become life-threatening was still too great.

The winter and spring of 1993/94 pretty much put our family life through a meat grinder. Afterwards, things were utterly different. Except for the rare visit out, I was confined to the house, and my mum had to stay at home to take care of me. We all became au fait with previously unfamiliar medical terms.

Mai had to learn how to clean my Broviac. This needed to be done twice a week. My skin would sting as she swabbed with an alcohol wipe the site where the catheter came out of my chest. Mum would then clean the tubes with another alcohol wipe, before cracking open a phial and drawing Heparin Lock Flush Solution (Hep-Lock) up into a syringe via a needle. She'd push the needle into one of the green bungs at the end of my Broviac, and pass the solution up through the line. When the first little tube had been flushed, the other two would get their turns. I still get shivers when I think of the cold sensation of the solution flowing beneath my skin.

Usually, a Broviac would be protected by sticking the tubes to the patient's chest with adhesive tape. There would also be a dressing covering the site where the tube exited the chest. We discovered shortly after my Broviac was inserted, however, that adhesive dressings and adhesive tape irritated the skin on my chest — they would both make me glow red with a rash. The hospital team tried several types of dressing, but each one wreaked havoc on my skin. In the end, my Broviac entry site was left uncovered. However, I still needed a substitute for the adhesive tape — if the Broviac tubes were not held in place somehow, there was a risk that a fall or other sudden movement could yank the entire apparatus from my body. My parents asked the hospital team if there was anything else that could be used to keep the cumbersome tubes up. The nurses suggested getting me a crop top.

So, one hugely embarrassing day, I trailed along behind my mother to Roches Stores in Blackrock, Co. Dublin. Mum strode into the girls' underwear section, while I hid behind a clothes rack a good distance away. Mai asked the shop assistant if we could have a look at some crop tops.

'Certainly,' the attractive young woman chimed. 'What size is your daughter?'

'Oh, no,' my mum laughed, 'it's for my son.'

There was a look of shock on the attendant's face as I sheepishly emerged from behind my clothes rack. She must have thought we were from some sort of bizarre cross-dressing family!

From that day forth, I began secretly wearing girls' undergarments beneath my t-shirts. I have to admit, though, I didn't find it as pleasurable as some men apparently do. My mum cut the frilly bits off the crop tops — so they at least looked a tad manlier.

It's strange. Yes, Fanconi anaemia changed our family life after

February 1994. But as we all got used to this new presence in our household, the panic that my parents had felt following my diagnosis faded.

For me, during those months I spent at home in the spring of '94, the idea of having a life-threatening illness had a streak of adventure in it. I hadn't come up against any real adversity. Taking an oxymethalone pill every day was no major deal. Having the Broviac felt weird, but it didn't really inconvenience me. I was a conscientious student, and being forced to stay out of school was upsetting, but our teacher sent me work, which I did in the house, so keeping up with my class wasn't a big problem. I missed the daily contact with my friends, but they were allowed call over on occasion—it wasn't as if I never got to see them.

Back then, I thought of Fanconi anaemia as something that made me unique, that set me apart from my peers. It was exciting to think I had a disease that no one else I knew had.

I recall, one day, paying a quick morning visit to BSP. I had come in basically just to let my classmates know how I was doing. I sat at the top of the room, in the teacher's chair, and fielded questions on my condition from subdued peers—a titillating power trip for my nine-year-old ego. Emma asked me what my chances of surviving into the future were.

Instead of trying to reassure her, my response was, 'I don't know that. My parents don't know that. Even my doctors don't know that.'

My routine at home during those days was not taxing. I got up mid-morning and gobbled a cooked breakfast (usually consisting of sausages, rashers, scrambled eggs and toast) provided by my mum, while watching the Cartoon Network. Then I did schoolwork for a few hours. In the evenings, I would draw comic strips or make stuff out of cardboard—do the random creative stuff I'd always done to amuse myself.

I never imagined the things that might happen to me because of this illness. I was just a kid whose life was a little different from his friends'.

Thanks to all the hours I spent watching the channel, I became quite familiar with some of the Cartoon Network's programmes. My favourite show was *Captain Planet and the Planeteers*. You probably remember the show. In it, five eco-conscious 'Planeteers' do battle with such fiendish 'eco-villains' as Hoggish Greedly, Dr Blight, and Looten Plunder. When the action becomes too much for the Planeteers to handle alone, they combine the powers from their magical rings — given to them by Gaia, the Spirit of the Earth — and summon the crystalline, eco-friendly superhero, Captain Planet.

I liked superheroes. I liked the idea of having the power to change things. Captain Planet's motto was 'The Power Is Yours!', implying that we could all be Planeteers, saving the world, if we chose to be. I used to imagine that our house was a hut on Hope Island, the Planeteers' home. I pretended I was one of those heroes with the magic rings. I had a toy ring, which had come with a Captain Planet action figure that my parents bought for me. I used to wear my plastic ring all day long.

Two months after I was prescribed oxymethalone, my blood counts were still low, and my immune system was nowhere near as strong as a healthy person's would be. The steroid was starting to have some positive effect — the petechiae had gone away, as had my spontaneous stomachaches. But I was well below the threshold at which the Crumlin team usually sent patients back into society. Dr Breatnach wanted me to live as normal a life as possible, but he could not see my condition improving much in the foreseeable future. So, he lowered the threshold.

In April 1994, after more than four months of being housebound, I returned to the Bray School Project.

I'd been gone for a term and a half, but rejoining my class wasn't awkward. I fitted easily back into the group of pals I'd hung around with previously. And, if I may say so, I remained a diligent pupil. No, not diligent — obsessive! I remember crying one day because I missed a few words in a spelling test as a teacher had come in to talk to me about something.

Life and death were not my main concerns back then. Apart from checkups in Crumlin every few weeks, Fanconi anaemia seemed a faraway problem. Third Class breezed into Fourth. And only my natural difficulty sleeping was keeping me awake at night.

3. Fartknocker

After Jess and I were diagnosed with FA in February '94, my parents made it their duty to find out as much as they could about the disorder. This led them to get in touch with the Fanconi Anemia Research Fund, Inc. — a non-profit, US-based corporation, founded in 1989 with the aim of furthering scientific research into FA, in the hope of improving treatments.

Mai and Des wanted to get involved in fundraising for both the FA Research Fund and Crumlin Hospital. They started out tentatively, holding a few pay-on-entry cheese and wine parties at our house, organising sponsored bag packs, etc. Then, in the summer of 1995 (between Fourth and Fifth Class for me), they got this wild notion that they wanted to do a fundraising climb up Mont Blanc.

Lying on the French border with Italy, Mont Blanc is the tallest of the Alps. Indeed, peaking almost five kilometres above sea level, it is the highest mountain in Western Europe.

Mum and Dad had always been avid hikers — a fact my sisters and I were acutely aware of, thanks to many frog-marches up Connemara hills. I suppose Mai and Des's love of hiking was where their interest in this expedition came from. My school friend Michael's father was one of very few qualified mountain guides in Ireland at the time. Michael's dad and a colleague of his agreed to take Mai, Des, and their posse of fundraising freaks up Mont Blanc. In the end, my parents, Michael's dad, the second guide, and two others made the trek.

It was in August '95 that Mai, Des, Ruth, Jess, and I boarded the ferry bound for France. As we drove onto the boat, I was feeling a little giddy. I had been to California when I was eleven months old, but, as you might expect, I didn't remember much of that trip. This fundraising expedition was going to be my first real foreign holiday.

Michael, his brothers, and his mum and dad were staying at a campsite in Argentière, in eastern France. We had rented an apartment nearby. The apartment was a cosy place with a balcony from which we had a glorious view of some local peak that cable cars were running up and down.

The apartment complex was right beside a glacial river. There was a concrete bridge over the river, and when you stood on the bridge and looked down into the grey, silt-filled water, you'd get a blast of cold air on your face. It was like stepping into one of those giant, walk-in freezers. There was a playground near our apartment, as well. However, all the play-things in this playground — the slide, the monkey bars, etc. — were made out of some kind of ultra-reflective, mirror-like metal. On hot days, these play-things became like hotplates, impossible to touch without burning yourself. It was brilliant — Michael, his brothers, my sisters, and I could go to the river and get frozen, and then go to the playground and get scorched!

We also had great fun with the apartment block's elevator. This elevator had the word 'fartknocker' graffitied inside it — a delightful word, the meaning of which I have yet to discover. We used the lift to cruise from floor to floor; on each floor, we would dash through the corridors like cats on speed. The lights in these corridors were on a sort of energy-saving timer system. Half the time, we'd be sprinting through the halls in complete darkness — that was the fun of it.

My parents spent some of the first week of our trip acclimatising for the trek to come. But Ruth, Jess, and I did get the opportunity to go on several breathtaking walks in the Alpine foothills with them. The heat was stifling, but the sights spectacular — mountain paths twisting through forests, decorated with beautiful flowers. And if you looked up, you'd see the peaks of the Alps, towering over the clouds, snow sparkling on their sides.

When my sisters and I weren't in the apartment block or on walks with Mai and Des, we could usually be found at Michael's campsite, or hanging around 'Le Yeti', a café-bar near our apartment which came complete with its own swimming pool. For me, 'hanging around' essentially meant sitting by the side of the pool, munching pizza. Because of my Broviac, I couldn't swim, so I had a good excuse to just lounge under the big umbrellas and tease Ruth by telling her that horse burgers were on the menus of all the local restaurants (horses were Ruth's favourite animals).

In the second week of our stay in eastern France, Mai, Des, and their two companions were led up Mont Blanc by Michael's dad and the other guide. They departed early on Wednesday. Despite suffering blinding headaches and constant vomiting all the way up, they reached the mountain's frozen peak on Thursday morning. By sunset on the same day, the team was back down, battered yet jubilant. Some side effects of the climb lasted a while, though.

One evening a day or two after the trek, Des, Ruth, Jess, and I were relaxing in the living area of the Argentière apartment — playing cards, reading, just generally amusing ourselves.

Suddenly, Mai came bounding down the spiral staircase from the bedrooms. 'Gather the children!' she called to Des. 'Gather the children! I'm dying! I'm dying!'

She had tried to take an anti-inflammatory pill for back pain, but had been unable to swallow it. The tablet was now lodged in her throat, and she was finding it quite hard to breathe.

Dutifully, we all pulled on our coats, and traipsed with Mum to the local doctor's surgery.

Mai went in to see the GP, wailing about the fact that she had just come down from Mont Blanc — wouldn't it be rather sad if she now died trying to swallow a pill!

The French doctor instantly knew what was wrong. Mum's throat had become swollen as a result of the altitude, and that's why the stubborn tablet had refused to go down.

So he cauterised her throat and the anti-inflammatory was dislodged. The pill slipped into her stomach, and that was the end of the drama.

As we were leaving the surgery, the GP told Mai that she was a lovely person with wonderful children. Mum smiled insanely and gave him a 'thumbs up', saying, 'Do they use this sign in France?'

The final week of our three-week French holiday that summer was spent in Paris. We did all the touristy stuff — were awed by the view from atop the Eiffel Tower, wandered around the museums, lost ourselves in Disneyland . . .

All told, Mai and Des's mad/brave expedition up Europe's highest peak raised over twenty thousand pounds for Fanconi Research and Our Lady's. A photograph of my parents at the summit still rests on our sitting room windowsill in Kilmac.

I came back from my first holiday abroad feeling terrific. I had dipped my toes in the wider world, and loved it. As I prepared to go into Fifth Class, I could believe that Fanconi anaemia was going to have little influence on my life.

But this was the calm. The storms were on their way.

4. A boy and his steroid

'You're not fat, Ben,' my father said to me. We were seated on opposite sides of our kitchen table, a green tablecloth dividing us; I was supposed to be on my way to bed. 'A boy your age needs far more calories than you take in every day.'

'Who says I need to eat more?!' I demanded. 'Everybody's different!'

'Yes, everybody's different,' my mum, who was sitting beside Des, responded. 'But you're not well. We think your brain might be affected by —'

'Don't be fucking stupid!' I lashed out, not letting Mai finish.

'Don't talk to me like that!' my mum hit back.

I didn't have to listen to this shite. I screamed at Mai and Des to leave me alone, and thundered out of the room.

The following morning, I was still furious. But I couldn't let my anger get in the way of my routine. After getting dressed, I marched into the kitchen and took the box of cornflakes from its cupboard. I carried the cornflakes over to the weighing scales, and shook out exactly thirty grams' worth—the 'typical serving size', according to the side of the box. I then tossed the flakes from the scales into a bowl. I went to the fridge, and removed the low fat milk. I found a measuring jug, and poured precisely one hundred and twenty-five millilitres of milk into the jug. I drenched my cereal with the milk, and sat down to eat.

My breakfast didn't disperse my anger. When I got to school, I stormed into the classroom, ignoring everyone around me. Sensing that something wasn't right, our teacher took me aside. He led me into what we termed the 'ninth classroom'—a room to which groups could be sent to study; extra books were kept in this room, and it contained a small kitchen area for cookery classes.

Our teacher ushered me into a chair, then sat down opposite me.

'Is there anything wrong, Ben?' he asked.

Of course, every member of the BSP staff knew that I had Fanconi anaemia, and they were all willing to help in whatever way they could.

But I was a big Fifth Class boy now. I didn't want any help from teachers. 'No, there's nothing wrong.'

'Because,' the teacher continued, 'you know you can talk to me if there is, and it won't go beyond me.' He added, 'And I know you'll be able to articulate your problems, because, you know, talking to you is different from talking to other children your age. It's almost like speaking to an adult. I couldn't try and hold this conversation with . . . Well, with some other members of your class.'

'Like—' I named the most notorious delinquent in our class.

'Well,' the teacher smiled, 'you named names. I didn't want to do that. Anyway,' he concluded, 'I'm here if you need me.'

'Thanks,' I managed. 'But I'm fine.'

And with that, we both left the room.

I felt relieved as I walked back to class. My teacher hadn't discovered my secret.

A couple of months before, I had been put on another steroid in addition to the oxymethalone — prednisolone. Dr Breatnach had prescribed me prednisolone in the hope of boosting my still-slacking energy levels.

Shortly after I started taking this new drug, however, I had decided I was fat.

Now, I'd always been a thin child. But, over time, the use of oxymethalone had given me a bloated appearance. I did look overweight. And I had made up my mind to do something about it. The desk in my room was now cluttered with 'healthy eating' magazines. An eleven-year-old boy, I had cut sweets and treats out of my diet completely.

I was constantly trying to think of new and innovative ways to burn calories. I was now doing my homework standing up rather than sitting down. At home, if I wanted to go to the kitchen, I would walk down the corridor to the bathroom, then back up again, before going to the kitchen. In school, like a kid possessed, I spent my lunch breaks pounding up and down the playground. My friends had tried to follow me at first. But I saw it as my mission to out-walk them. In the end, I left them behind.

The bell rang. It was twenty to three — school was over for the day. I began to put my books into my bag. The guy sitting beside me, a good friend, turned to me. 'You look different to the way you looked before,' he said out of the blue. 'I can see all the bones in your face.'

'Thanks,' I said, and meant it.

I smiled. It had been a good day. I'd successfully concealed my problems from my teacher, and my friends obviously thought I was getting thinner.

I went outside to the sunshine. My mum was waiting for me in her red car. I opened the door and got in.

Most of the journey home went by in silence.

But then my mum said, 'You need to apologise for your attitude last night, Ben.'

I didn't say anything.

'Ben?'

Nothing.

'Ben?'

'Go fuck yourself.'

Mai slammed some sheets of paper down on the table in front of me. She'd been in my room, and had found these sheets hidden under my bed. Scrawled on the sheets were elaborate sets of sums that I had used to work out my daily calorific intake.

'What the fuck were you doing in my fucking room?!' I demanded.

I looked furiously at Mai, then at Des. Once again, the two parents had sat me down at the kitchen table for a 'talk'. Just a few days previously, they'd tried to tell me that I should eat more food. Now they were going through my private stuff! I'd managed to survive the whole day without eating anything except a banana and a packet of popcorn—and now I had to put up with this bullshit!

Mai ignored my question.

'This has got to stop,' she said. 'You have to eat something before you go to bed.'

'No!' I screeched. I was not going to lose my wonderful low-calorie day.

'Well,' Des said, 'you have to drink a glass of milk, at least.'

'Fuck off,' I said.

But Mai and Des threatened punishment. I had no choice but to drink the milk.

Once the glass was empty, I ran into my room and slammed the door. No one understood me. Why the hell couldn't I be allowed to live my own life?

I opened my cupboard, took out my turquoise tennis racquet, and unzipped and removed its cover. I hit myself over the head with the racquet's hard metal edge. I struck myself until my brain was abuzz with pain and confusion.

Then I took the chair from underneath my desk and flung it at the opposite wall, screaming fiercely.

I collapsed onto my bed and into tears. I lay there for hours, crying into the palms of my hands.

The next day, I wandered into the school grounds in a bleary-eyed daze. BSP had a decent-sized playground, the main feature of which was a tarmacadam basketball court. Most dry mornings, in the time leading up to nine o'clock and the start of lessons, students could be seen playing around this area, venting their energy. And every morning, at the strike of nine, a bell would ring out, and each pupil would line up with his or her classmates. The teachers would then lead their classes into the mild-yellow-coloured BSP building.

On this morning, as I trudged across the basketball court to the place where Fifth-Classers queued up, a friend innocently called from behind me, 'Hi, Ben!'

And I completely lost it. I turned around, ran to him, jumped on his back and started pummelling him.

After a few seconds, I fell to the ground, exhausted. My friend did not retaliate. He just drifted away.

This was the beginning of a vicious, almost uncontrollably aggressive me.

I hit my parents when they asked me to do chores — my dad and my mum. I hit them when they didn't ask me to do anything. I just clenched my fists and punched.

My young sisters weren't free from my violence either. Des and Mai could not leave me alone in a room with Ruth and Jess, because of a real fear that I'd seriously hurt them.

My temper would come and pass, but I was always wired, ready to strike. When I flew off the handle, I became borderline psychotic. My face would turn purple, the veins poking out on my forehead. If

I was at home, I often ran out to our front yard. Then I would stop, build myself up, and sprint up and down the garden as fast as I could. On more than one occasion, I kicked my mum's car with such force that it had to be taken to a panel beater to repair the dents.

This behaviour went on for months. My parents, convinced the prednisolone was the cause, asked Dr Breatnach if it was really necessary to keep me on the second steroid. He thought it was. My blood counts had not performed particularly well when I was only on oxymethalone. Now that I was taking prednisolone, they were looking a lot better. Yes, developing an obsession with food and becoming uncharacteristically aggressive were two known side effects of prednisolone. But was getting rid of these side effects worth risking my life over?

You may consider it an odd statement, but St John's Ward in Crumlin Hospital was always a beautiful place to me. There were the dull blue floors and the bland beige walls, of course. But mounted on those walls were images of innocence and hope—stunningly colourful drawings by many patients, and framed collages of photos featuring bald boys and girls meeting beaming celebrities. The waiting area, and the conservatory in the High Dependency Unit that I mentioned before, were usually littered with toys. But there was one place in the ward which naturally had more toys than anywhere else—the playroom.

I remember sitting in this playroom in early summer 1996, at a small table in one of the corners, talking to a dietician. She was attempting to convince me that it was okay to consume in moderation the foods I enjoyed but was denying myself. What a curious sight it must have been: a professional dietician urging an eleven-year-old boy to eat pizzas, burgers, chocolate, and crisps!

Taking prednisolone for nearly a year had resulted in a major improvement in my blood counts, and Dr Breatnach had decided the time was right to begin weaning me off the drug. The theory was that the prednisolone had kick-started the oxymethalone into action, and now that this had happened, I could be weaned off the prednisolone safely.

With the second steroid on the way out, the healing process had begun.

I remember the dietician saying to me that afternoon in '96, 'Pizza is particularly good, I think, because you've got all different food types there—bread, tomatoes, cheese; then with toppings you can have meat, or more vegetables. You see, Ben, we don't look at any one-off meal, but at a person's diet as a whole, to judge how what they eat affects their weight.'

It was a lesson I needed to learn. And with the help of that dietician, I did learn it. Once I was off the prednisolone, a more balanced attitude toward food crept into my mind. I lost the intense interest in counting calories, but I remained concerned with healthy eating. For over a year after I stopped taking the steroid, I still wouldn't treat myself to sweets.

With the prednisolone gone, I settled down into my more placid self again, as well. It was like finding a friend who had gone AWOL.

I never really talked to anyone about that period of my life when I was anorexic enough to be a danger to myself, and angry enough to be a danger to my friends and family. Throughout the period itself, I was pretty much immune to all attempts by those close to me to pierce through my armour of rage.

I recall one sunny evening during that time, though, out in our back garden at home, yelling at Dad over something stupid. He looked at me, sadly, and told me he didn't think I was turning out to be a good person. I remember that comment cut through my fury and my obsession, and reached my heart like the sharpest blade.

After the confrontation, I went into the house. I was lost; I didn't know what to do, so I mechanically went to the bathroom to wash my hands. I let the water slip over them, and then I turned off the tap. I left the bathroom and walked halfway down the corridor. Suddenly, I stopped. Did I wash my hands or just imagine that I did? I questioned myself. I returned to the bathroom, and let the water run over my hands once more. I again walked down the corridor. Idiot! You'll need to clean them better than that! I turned around to wash my hands another time.

This pattern continued until I'd washed my hands ten times. I was stuck; I'd nowhere else to go. The pattern was all I had. Every time I washed my hands, I convinced myself I hadn't washed them properly.

And as the water fell through my fingers, all I wanted to do was forget who I was.

5. Emma

From the age of eleven to twelve upwards, most boys and girls are in for a turbulent and exciting time, what with hormones flinging themselves all over the place. As we made our way through primary school, the knowledge I and most of my friends possessed about sex was limited, to say the least. Back in Second Class, one of my pals insisted to me that 'condom' was another word for 'shit'. I thought 'condom' was some kind of cream one put on one's private parts. I remember, I learned what an orgasm is while looking up the word 'organism' in the dictionary. Oh, the innocence!

This youthful naivety was royally smashed, however, during Fifth Class, when my classmates and I were shown a grotesquely explicit Sexual Education video. The programme followed a mommy and a daddy as they walked around their house, naked. The camera offered us close-ups of the daddy's penis and the mommy's vagina. The video then cut to a rather stiff animation, and the female narrator stoically offered this description of sexual intercourse: 'And then the man inserts his penis into the woman's vagina, and it feels very nice.' Indeed. But for whom?

Now, I'm not saying it was because of the Sex Ed video, but it does seem a bit of a coincidence that it was around the same time as we viewed this charming programme, that males and females in our class became interested in one another in ways which went beyond friendship. Couples started forming among my friends toward the end of Fifth Class. It wasn't until Sixth Class, however, that we preteens began seriously 'going out' with members of the opposite sex — i.e. holding hands with them in the playground.

As I went into Sixth Class, things were a lot different for me from the way they'd been over the previous year. During the summer holidays of 1996, much changed for the better. The oxymethalone started to carry the weight of my counts on its own. My dose was lowered; I lost that bloated look. Then, my Broviac was removed, and I no longer had to wear girls' underwear. With my checkups down to once a month, and no bone marrow transplant anywhere in sight, Dr

Breatnach felt taking out the catheter was for the best. Most Broviacs, anyway, are put in for about a year — nearly three years was a good run.

During the summer of '96, I also found something which gave me more joy than anything had in a long time. Some people discover God, religion; I discovered . . . Michael Jackson.

One afternoon while travelling in the car with my parents, I heard 'Earth Song' on the radio. Over the previous couple of years, my love of *Captain Planet and the Planeteers* had made me quite environmentally conscious. When I heard Jackson's 'Earth Song' for the first time, its 'love the planet' message resonated with me. A few weeks later, Des and I were in the Golden Discs record shop in Bray, and he offered to buy me any album I wanted. I chose MJ's two-CD, greatest-hits-and-new-material collection, *HIStory*.

That's how my Michael Jackson fanaticism took seed. I'd never had much of an interest in music before then. I had collected a few CDs over the preceding two years, but I was never sure whether I liked any of the songs on them or not. They just seemed to be the kinds of things my friends listened to.

From the moment I put on *HIStory*, though, and heard classics ranging from 'Billie Jean' and 'Bad' to 'Stranger in Moscow' — things were different. I knew what kind of music I liked.

Over time, I acquired other MJ CDs. I bought copies of all his adult solo albums, and copies of most of his work with the Jacksons and the Jackson 5. I purchased his videos, and later his DVDs. His short films were mesmerising, his live performances electrifying. And something about Michael's voice sang to every part of me. It became my refuge — that voice which is one of the greatest, most versatile musical instruments in the world today. Whenever I felt lost, sad, angry, or alone, there was some Michael Jackson track I could put on that would make me feel known, make me feel understood.

As I entered Sixth Class, the King of Pop's music was what was making me happy — while all my friends were turning to the opposite sex to get their thrills.

I wasn't completely out of step with my pals, though. Sixth Class made my attention turn to girls, too. Well, one girl — a member of my class whom I had always been particularly fond of.

Who can say where these things really come from, but I suppose I was attracted to Emma because she was everything I was not, and, consequently, everything I admired: glowing, outgoing, full of life and fun, beautiful. She was gracefully slender; she had shining, neck-length light brown hair, and the purest white skin you ever saw.

Emma was also someone who had always been kind to me, especially during the troubles of Third Class. While I was in hospital, she wrote me one letter in which she scribbled the words 'I MISS YOU!' in very large capitals.

Emma and I both loved drama, as well. During Second Class, we starred together in a production of a play based on the mythological life of Fionn mac Cumhaill. I had the role of Fionn, and Emma was my wife. We had tremendous fun with that play. When we staged it for the BSP parents, my mum came, and she brought with her my two-year-old cousin. In the middle of the show, the brat sprang from Mai's arms, ran to me, and started pulling off my fake beard, screeching, 'Ben! Ben!' That spoiled the performance somewhat.

The 'Fionn' play wasn't the only one I starred in with Emma. In Third Class, before I got sick, Emma, her twin sister Michelle, and I used to make up our own little sketches, and improvise them in front of our classmates.

In the spring term of Sixth Class, this interest in Emma, and the desire of my classmates to match-make, somehow led to me writing her a letter in which I told her how I felt. The letter was passed on to Emma by a friend.

Writing to a girl was something I could do; actually going up and asking her out, was not.

Emma's response also came in written form. In her missive, she wrote, 'Ben, I am replying to your letter. I can't blame you for fancying me (joke)!!! Let's not talk about it again as I'm finding it hard to do English with you. Thanks for fancying me, I'm flattered.'

It was a polite brush-off. I picked myself up after it, and carried on with my life as if my first romantic hopes had not been dashed against jagged rocks.

A few weeks later, I was in the ninth classroom with my reading group. We were rehearsing a radio drama, *The Invisible Man*, which we were going to record and play for the rest of the class. I was annoyed, because the production's director had just snootily criticised my pronunciation of the word 'heard'.

Suddenly, I was surprised by someone tapping me on the small of my back.

I turned around to see who had tapped me. It was Emma.

'Do you remember Third Class, when we did all those plays?' she asked.

I nodded.

'I used to fancy you then.'

I didn't know how to respond. 'You used to touch my hair a lot,' I said.

'Will you come to Jackie's disco with me?' Emma asked. 'Jackie's disco' was a party which had been arranged to celebrate the birthdays of four members of our class, including Emma and Michelle. Everyone from Sixth Class was going.

I couldn't say anything. I was astounded. Emma wanted to take me to her own birthday party! I just stood and nodded.

In April 1997, Emma and I went to the disco—my first disco! The party was held in Jackie's house, about a mile away from my house, in Kilmacanogue. In the days leading up to the party, I bought hair gel for the first time, and tried it out on my brown locks (those furious white curls had disappeared some years earlier). I also displayed an active interest in clothes shopping for the first time, and my mum took me to buy a new black jacket, black t-shirt, and black jeans, especially for the disco.

I arrived at Jackie's house fashionably late on the evening of the party, with a friend in tow. Jackie's parents had hired a DJ for the occasion, and their living room was decked with disco lights. The place looked exactly like what I imagined a disco to be.

I had brought presents for the four birthday girls. I was standing in the doorway of the 'disco room' when I handed Emma her gift. She thanked me, unwrapped it, smiled, then kissed me lightly on the cheek. I grinned nervously.

Even though I was there as her 'date', I didn't really hang out with Emma at the party that night. I spent most of the time standing beside the tables at the back of the living room; these tables were loaded with crisp- and sweet-filled plastic bowls, and I would watch spots of green and red disco-light spin across the crisps and the sweets and the bowls. Once during the evening, my friends pushed me towards Emma. She looked at me, wondering what I was going to do.

I just smiled apologetically, and wandered off.

In the wake of Jackie's disco, it seemed that Emma and I were 'going out'. But I still didn't spend much time with her. I wanted to, but spending time with her meant hanging around with her friends, or engaging in the holding of hands or other such intimacies. I desperately desired to be with Emma. But I was terrified of physical contact. It was far easier to have us 'going out' in name only.

Yet I was willing to do whatever I could to stay in my 'relationship' with this amazing girl. One bright spring morning, as we stood in the brown-carpeted Sixth Class classroom, Michelle informed me that Emma was 'drawing a line'. Unless I offered some sign of my interest in her by the end of the day, she was going to 'break it off' with me. For hours, I fretted. How could I display my passion? I knew I couldn't pen another letter, that would never work.

When the bell rang for home time, I made sure I left the classroom before anyone else. I waited just outside the classroom doors, leaning against a cupboard in the 'shared area' between Fifth Class and Sixth. A tide of eleven-, twelve-, and thirteen-year-olds gushed by; everyone had a schoolbag on his or her back, everyone was chatting and laughing, everyone was happy that another five and a half hours of lessons were over.

As Emma passed me, I moved forward till I was right beside her. Then, ever so briefly, I let my lips touch her perfect, cloud-white cheek.

Michelle, who was behind Emma, cooed, 'Awwww.' Some of our other classmates swapped glances. But Emma said nothing. And neither did I. I lifted my schoolbag off the floor, and went home.

This gesture on my part, however, was not enough to salvage what I had with Emma. The next morning, Michelle told me that the 'relationship' was over.

Our twelve-year-olds' romance had lasted all of three days.

It was a Bray School Project tradition that, every year, Sixth Class departed on a three-day trip to the largest of the Aran Islands, Inishmore.

One morning in the middle of May 1997, I awoke at 5.45 a.m. I think it was the earliest I'd ever been awake. I had to be at BSP by 6.30. Our class was due to get a bus to Heuston Station, Dublin. There, we would catch a train to Galway City. From Galway City we would make our way to Rossaveal, and then take a ferry to Aran.

Three BSP teachers came with us to Inishmore, including the man who'd taught me during Fifth Class. He brought a camcorder, and made a souvenir videotape of the trip. On the ferry on the way to the island, on that tape, some friends and I can be seen pretending to get sick over the side of the boat. I thought this was a great way to keep the camera on me.

There was also another adult who came with us to Inishmore that May: my mum. A teacher herself, Mai sometimes did substitute work at BSP. But she was asked to come on the Aran trip so she could keep an eye on me. If I got sick, they'd need someone who knew what to do.

When our ferry docked at the harbour in Kilronan, the 'capital' of the Aran Islands, each member of my class grabbed his or her luggage, and we all bounded up to the green- and red-coloured hostel where we would be staying. Most of us would be in rooms with our friends.

Stretching between our hostel and the harbour was a sandy, seaweed-flecked beach. Behind the beach there were B&Bs, pubs, places to rent bicycles.

That evening, after we'd eaten, almost everyone in our class went down to the beach between the hostel and the harbour. The sky was a whitish grey, and little droplets of rain were speckling the light sand with dark spots. But the dull weather was not enough to dim the holiday atmosphere each of us felt.

I was standing on my own, smiling and watching my classmates enjoy themselves, when Emma approached me. She told me that she needed to get something off her chest, and asked if we could talk.

We began to stroll side by side along the shoreline.

'Ben,' she started, 'I've always sort of fancied you . . .'

My heart leapt.

' . . . as a friend.'

And sank again.

Grunts were about all I managed, as Emma continued to explain why she thought we should just be friends. In her speech, there was nothing that I didn't know already. But, I guess, even after we'd 'split up', I'd still held a tiny hope that there could be more between us.

After our talk, I didn't feel like staying on the beach. I went and found the four adults, who were seated in an outbuilding which served as a kitchen-cum-dining area for the hostel we were staying in. There was a bottle of wine open on their table, and the quartet of grownups was debating where the end of the universe might be. 'I think it's out past Dun Aengus!' one teacher said loudly, laughing.

I asked my mum, and my own class teacher, if I could be allowed to go for a walk. Thankfully, Mai and my teacher gave me permission to amble off. They urged me to try and find the aforementioned end of the universe.

I moseyed along the water's edge, away from Aran's 'capital'. After a while, I came to a stony strand, different from the sandy one in Kilronan. All the stones were wonderfully smooth, and they got smaller and smaller the nearer they were to the sea. There was a little wooden hut perched on the stones. The hut's door was missing, and fishing nets and lobster pots were spilling out.

I sat down among the rocks and pebbles. I covered my face with my hands, and began to softly sing Michael Jackson's lonely song 'Stranger in Moscow'. The rain felt like mist against my skin.

I wasn't quite sure what I wanted from Emma. But just being friends wasn't it.

The remainder of the Aran trip was understandably an anticlimax, after that first night.

The following morning, everyone in the class except for me set out on a cycle tour of the island. I was forbidden from riding a bike because, if I fell off, the cuts and bruises I might receive could lead to a dangerous level of bleeding.

So, my mother and I hopped on a minibus, and joined everyone else at the ancient cliff-top fort of Dun Aengus. There, my classmates and I munched our packed lunches. Then, we were each given an opportunity to gaze over the edge of the hundred-metre-high cliff at the churning waters below. One at a time, we all lay flat on the ground at the edge of the cliff, our heads jutting out into the air, while two teachers gripped our legs to ensure that no accidents took place. I remember we were told not to spit down into the raging waves. To paraphrase a pal of mine—I'm not sure what the point of that instruction was. It's not as if there were people swimming below!

On the day after the cycle tour, BSP's Class of '97 deserted

Inishmore. On my Fifth Class teacher's film of the trip, I can be heard saying on the ferry on the way home, 'Yes! We're off that cursed island!'

Our school life went back to normal once the Aran trip was over. However, my soap opera with Emma was not entirely complete. Two days after we returned from Inishmore, I was hanging out with friends in the schoolyard at lunch break. Emma sauntered up to me, a posse of her own pals in tow.

'Will you go out with me?' she asked, looking straight at me.

You must be thinking what I was thinking: What the fuck? Nonetheless, if the girl who still occupies your daydreams asks you to be her man, even if you're mightily confused, you don't turn her down. So I said 'Yes.'

The birthday party of another classmate was held in Blackrock a few days later. My dad drove me to this classmate's house; I pressed the doorbell and was let in by the birthday girl. I was taken to the kitchen-cum-living area, where many of my friends were already lounging. Current pop tunes were blaring from a sound system, flooding the room with thumping four by four beats.

I spent most of that evening with Emma. We didn't say much to each other; I didn't know what to say. But I liked just sitting beside her.

At one point, I left the kitchen-cum-living area to go to the toilet. On my way back, I passed Michelle. I told her I didn't know why Emma had said she simply wanted to be friends with me, and had then asked me out again.

'Well,' Michelle was at a loss. 'She really likes you, Ben. She told me, she almost loves you, like.'

I hadn't expected that answer.

I returned to Emma feeling reassured and elated, and we watched as several other members of our class played spin-the-bottle.

When the fun of snogging random people had been exhausted, someone put some romantic music on, and all the couples stood up to slow-dance.

Emma curled her arms around me, and I wrapped my arms around her, and we moved together in blissful, effortless circles.

I had always been loved. I had my mum and dad, my sisters, and many brilliant friendships. But whatever this thing with Emma was, it was the first relationship that wasn't part of the background scenery of my life — the first relationship I didn't take for granted. And in those few minutes, holding Emma's body gently against my chest, I felt more than just a person unto myself. I felt a part of someone else's existence. I felt important to someone.

The bright days of May 1997 became the sunny days of June 1997. And the end of my six years at the Bray School Project loomed ever nearer, like an unstoppable train rattling rapidly down the track toward my station. With this in mind, I began to wonder what would happen to Emma and me once we moved to different secondary schools. I worried about keeping in contact with her. I worried about keeping in contact with all my friends, but I knew I at least wouldn't need an excuse to stay in touch with my male pals. I might need something that I could use as an excuse for staying in touch with Emma.

I had always been creative. At the age of seven, I wrote little plays, and performed them every Saturday morning for my parents and infant sisters. In Third Class, I made up a quiz game called 'The Questionator', and forced my hapless classmates to participate in it. In Fourth Class, I ran an exclusive club — two of my friends were the only other members. I named our club the 'MegaClub', and I wrote a club newsletter. We used to hold secret meetings in my tree house, and in the tree house of one of my pals.

My latest idea — the idea that I hoped would keep me in touch with Emma — was to start a new club, and invite all my friends to become members. This club would have its own magazine which I would edit, and which my friends would write for. If we were all running this little community, my BSP pals and I — Emma and I — would stay in contact by default.

Having come up with the mental blueprints, the only thing I now needed was a name for my club.

My dad had a friend, Terry O'Driscoll. Terry used to write crazy poems, such as this one about a 'Littal Buhrd':

> Oh, *Littal Buhrd*,
> *Of no name*,
> *I felt a twinge*

As I took aim.
I said,
'My God! I am de pits!'
But
BOOM! BOOM!
Ha! Ha!
You're in bits!

I loved Terry's poems, and he would write them out for me on sheets of paper. After the poems, he'd write, 'TM & © Nottwell'. Terry claimed he got the idea for this from something my sister Jess said. Mum had been asking Jess to do her chores, and Jess had moaned, 'I'm not well, Mai!' Terry thought 'Nottwell' would be a good name for a company—and I thought it would be a good name for a club. So, at the end of May '97, showing reckless disregard for all known intellectual property rights, I invited about a dozen of my BSP friends to join the 'Nottwel Club'. One night, I stayed up late, making membership cards out of green cardboard and contact paper. The next day, I tried to foist them upon my pals.

The initial response was mixed. Emma told me that she was too busy to let something like my club into her life right now. I tried to pretend I wasn't devastated.

'Did you just expect everyone would want to join?' Michelle asked me.

'No,' I lied.

'Why did you make membership cards for everyone already then?'

'I . . . Well, just in case everyone wanted to join.'

By lunch break on that particular day, however, attitudes had changed. Once Emma and the other naysayers discovered that I was offering free sweets to those who joined, they all agreed to become members of my club. And they even became excited about it. Michelle made Nottwel pens by taping the word 'Nottwel' onto biros; Emma wrote a poem about how great the club was. A week after my handing out the membership cards, Nottwel produced its first zine, *The Fush Monthly* #1.

'Fush' was another term Terry had coined. I think it was originally intended as a euphemism for a similar-sounding four-letter word. However, 'fush' took on a life of its own, and came to be used by my friends and me in multiple contexts—it could mean whatever we liked. We would even go around saying 'May the Fush be with you!' to each other.

Well, no, actually, it was just me who said that.

Writing the mag was a bit of fun, but I also wanted to entertain my friends and encourage them to keep in contact with one another once we left primary school. When the mag was finished, I gave it to Des so he could make copies with the photocopier in his office. I took these copies into school and distributed them among my classmates.

TFM #1 was a milestone literary achievement. It included such features as short comic strips plagiarised from a Disney magazine, and an interview with the incomparable Ben Murnane!

After the Nottwel Club came into existence, I wanted to do something special to celebrate its founding, and to mark the forthcoming passage of my classmates and myself from primary school.

I asked my parents if I could host a party at our house in mid-June. I invited my entire class, along with some of the BSP teaching staff.

At family barbecues as a younger kid, I often used to pretend I was Buddy Holly. I'd mime the rock'n'roll singer's songs while wearing my dad's old glasses and strumming on my toy guitar. For my farewell-to-Sixth-Class party, I longed to act the pop star once again. I wanted the centre-piece of the night to be a performance of Michael Jackson's 'Thriller' by me and Emma.

After I'd handed out the party invitations in school, I sidled up to Emma and asked her if she would be willing to participate in my proposed double act. She said she would. Michelle was eavesdropping on our conversation, and she turned to me with a patronising look, and scoffed, 'You know, Ben, no one likes Michael Jackson.'

I thought about saying, 'Well, he's the biggest selling artist of all time, so there must be a fault in your theory somewhere.' But I didn't say that. I just smiled, and defiantly told Michelle that I didn't care if no one liked MJ.

During the two weeks between the issuing of invitations and the evening of the party, I must have viewed the fourteen-minute 'Thriller' film dozens of times. I tirelessly studied Michael's moves, copying for my own performance the ones I could, discarding the others. I scrawled my choreography down on sheets of paper, and tried to memorise it and put it into practice while listening to the song. I rehearsed in our sitting room at home. Sometimes, my two sisters would stand in the doorway, observing and giggling as I thrust my fists into the air and twirled on my feet. I let them laugh away. I was going to be Michael Jackson for a night, and I was going to dance with a beautiful girl.

In the 'Thriller' video, MJ and his female friend emerge from a cinema and quarrel for a brief time before Michael begins to sing. I wanted to replicate this scene in my own performance. I recorded the song onto a new tape, leaving about two minutes 'blank' before the track began. This would give Emma and me time to row.

On a balmy summer's eve, classmates and teachers arrived at my family's Kilmacanogue home. My dad barbecued burgers, sausages, and chicken, and everybody sat eating and enjoying each other's company. Then, as darkness slunk across the sky, I gathered my friends around our newly constructed patio.

Emma came up to me. 'What am I supposed to do?' she asked.

And then suddenly it hit me. I should have rehearsed the thing with Emma! I had practised my 'Thriller' dance moves endlessly on my own, but the two of us had not rehearsed anything together.

'Just react to what I do,' I vaguely advised. 'And look scared. Oh, and at the end of the song, when the evil laughter starts, fall down dead.'

I turned to my audience. 'Good evening, everybody,' I began. 'Now, as most of you will know, Michael Jackson's *Thriller* is the biggest selling album of all time.' I went on to explain a little about the performance Emma and I were going to put on. I was finishing up, 'Now, we don't have the King of Pop here tonight,' when one friend shouted, 'But we do have Ben!'

I grinned. 'Exactly.'

And with that, I gestured to Des to push 'play' on the tape deck.

Emma and I began our argument, as if we had just left the cinema. She was scared, she told me. 'It's only a movie,' I replied.

We concluded our verbal combat, and Emma stepped back, expecting the music to start.

But I had left too much 'blank time' at the beginning of the cassette!

I paced around the patio for a few seconds, waiting for the eerie footsteps and evil howls to signal the song's start.

When they were not to be heard, I figured I'd better do something.

I began to sing MJ's recent number one hit, 'Blood on the Dance Floor', replacing the name of the girl in the chorus, 'Susie', with 'Emma'.

Then: Oh thank God, I thought, as the opening sounds of 'Thriller' seeped into the air.

And from that point on, I just danced. I tried to tempt Emma towards me, but she'd slip away, frightened. We both played our parts well.

At the first cackle of Vincent Price's maniacal laughter, Emma dutifully collapsed onto the ground, dead. I glanced frantically around, then sprinted off into the back garden, as the creaky door's closing signalled the end of the song.

When I returned to the party, my friends seemed surprised.

'Wow!' said one. 'I didn't know you could dance like that!'

'That was amazing!' commented another.

'You should have moonwalked into her,' was the only nugget of criticism offered.

A few minutes later, as I strutted into the house through the French doors, intending to pour myself a cooling drink, I passed a pair of teachers who were sitting in deckchairs by the patio's edge. The two teachers were talking about the fact that Emma and Michelle looked very alike, even though they were not identical twins. One asked the other, 'Which one was that dancing with Ben? I can never tell the difference.'

The second teacher glanced at me playfully, and said, 'I think Ben knows the difference!'

After my celebratory barbecue and my heart-stopping 'Thriller' performance, the 'End Of Primary School' train really was almost at my station. The final day of term is usually a Friday, and 1997 — in this sense at least — was a very usual year. As our last day at BSP approached, nobody in my class was thinking about work anymore. We were all giddily looking forward to our chance to take part in another Bray School Project tradition — the Sixth Class disco.

The event was held on the Wednesday of our final week. That night, I was hardly able to eat my dinner, so excited were the nerves fluttering in my stomach. I arrived at the school just after eight o'clock, sporting the same black jeans, black t-shirt, and black jacket that I had worn to Jackie's party. My hair was rendered immovable by gel.

The assembly hall in BSP had been converted into a nightclub for the evening — disco ball, coloured lights, contracted DJ — the only thing missing was alcohol. But, for a nominal sum, soft drinks and chocolatey snacks could be purchased from a teacher manning a makeshift concession stand.

For the first few songs of the night, I drifted on the sidelines. But after the Jacksons' 'Blame it on the Boogie' was played, I felt more at ease. Classmates coaxed me into the fray, and we giggled as we tried to copy one another's dance moves.

A brief while passed, and then I spotted Emma. She noticed me, too, and ran to where I was standing. We held each other beneath the flashing lights. I leaned forward to shout something into her ear over the excruciating noise.

And before I knew what was happening, her lips were on mine; her tongue was in my mouth, twirling softly around.

And then she was gone.

What the hell? I opened my eyes after our kiss only to glimpse Emma running toward the edge of the hall, back to the safety of her friends.

I didn't see her again for the rest of the night.

The following day, Thursday, was a normal school day. Throughout those five and a half hours, Emma managed to avoid talking to me, even going near me.

I had no prior experience and was caught off guard; I'm willing to accept that my attempt at a kiss may have been utterly awful.

Emma's kiss had come out of nowhere; in the confusion of every-thing that had gone back and forth between us, it was the strongest piece of evidence I had that she really felt something for me. I guess maybe I was confused or hurt or angry, because Emma was now ig-noring me. But I don't remember any of that. I remember being high from my first kiss.

As I daydreamed in class that Thursday, the penultimate day of my time in primary school, I thought about writing something beau-tiful for Emma, something she would always remember.

Then an idea struck me. Why not make a card for each member of my class, and make some cards for the BSP staff as well? These were the people who'd made all those cards for me when I was in hospital, after all.

I worked through Thursday night, till one o'clock on Friday morning, scribbling 'thank you' and 'farewell' messages to friends and teachers alike. And there was one message that I spent longer on than any of the others — I wanted to write something that would really touch Emma.

I ambled shadow-eyed into BSP at 9 a.m. on Friday, my last day with the class I had come to love. There was no schoolwork to be done. I handed out my cards, and a few friends gave me parting gifts in return. Michelle presented me with the cover of *The Fush Monthly* #1 in a frame. She said it was a gift from her and her sister.

Some moments went by. Then, as I stood lost in conversation with a group of friends, I felt a familiar tap on the small of my back.

I turned, and there was Emma. In her left hand, she was clutching my card. Her eyes were red, and tears glistened on her pretty white cheeks.

She tossed her arms around me, and I held her close.

Many others cried that morning. As a class, we had got on so well together, and now we were to be split up forever. In those few hours, it seemed as though our lives would never recover.

We spent the remainder of the school day jotting what we hoped would be unforgettable messages on one another's t-shirts and copybooks. At home time, there were hugs and goodbyes all round. I looked about me, but couldn't spot Emma. Then I saw her, on the other side of the room. She was talking to Jackie, and I could hear what she was saying. Wet streaks were staining her beautiful face.

'But what if I never see Ben again?' she said.

'Of course you'll see him again,' Jackie soothed. 'You can come up to me and we'll go and see him together.'

I hadn't cried during school that day. But as I reached home, I felt all my sadness make its way to my eyes. Clear droplets started slipping down my cheeks.

I went into our sitting room, and slotted my copy of the Aran videotape into the VCR. I sat in my usual seat in front of the TV. My eyes were raw and blurred from the tears.

I watched my friends and myself play and smile and laugh—we were oblivious to the parting that was oh-so-fast approaching us. And as I watched, I couldn't but wonder if I was crying for everybody in the video whom I would miss. Or if I was crying for just that one person whom I knew I would miss most of all.

6. Firsts

The question hadn't come from a friend, but a guy I didn't know: 'Do you put hair gel in your eyebrows?'

'No,' I answered, trying to laugh. I was standing outside a classroom, waiting for lunch break to end so I could go inside. I was now a First Year student at St Andrew's College, Booterstown, Co. Dublin.

'Because,' this fellow continued, 'you've got all these white bits in your eyebrows — looks like dried gel.'

'No, it's just my face,' I said, pointing to my forehead, 'it's . . '

'Yeah, it's horrible.'

'I know.'

Starting secondary school had been tough. I had to get up earlier, come home later, study more. This was no different from the rest of the First Year students, of course. But then, my haemoglobin was less than half that of any other St Andrew's newcomer.

I was exhausted.

I remember, every morning, before our class roll was called, there would be other kids running around the desks or hopping up and down on brown and grey plastic chairs. All I felt like doing was returning to my bed for a very long time.

I spent so many of my lessons on autopilot. Often, at the end of a school day, I would sit at my desk at home, look at the notes I'd taken in class, and not recall a thing about the context in which they'd been written.

And then there was my skin problem. I don't know whether it was brought on by stress or what, but around the middle of First Year, the skin on my face became horridly flaky. This, combined with my tired, sunken eyes, made me ripe for teasing by my schoolmates.

I was no stranger to skin problems. One morning during Fourth Class, at the age of ten, I had woken up to spy a little spot on one of my cheeks. As the days went by, my face had become more and more studded with spots, until the entire thing was lumpy, red, and slick with grease. I was taken to a dermatologist in Crumlin, who said she'd never seen acne so bad in one so young. My favourite little white pills, oxymethalone, were blamed for the outbreak.

My face had once been too greasy; now it was the opposite. It looked like an obscene white jigsaw puzzle; the skin flaked apart at my lightest touch. My forehead was especially bad. I would put on moisturiser before going to school, but by the middle of the day my forehead would again be parched and cracked.

I hated my skin, my face. It was two years since I had been taken off prednisolone, but some of the old attitudes were beginning to slip back: the obsession with my appearance, the self-loathing . . . I wanted to break all the mirrors in our house, so I wouldn't be able to look at myself. I used to come home from school, look in my mirror, and want to smash my face against my reflection. Maybe shards of glass could bleed this thing out of me.

It's funny, sometimes, how something can be two opposing things at once. Beginning secondary school was hard because of the tiredness and my skin and the teasing that came with them. But it was also exciting: taking on new subjects, making new friends, finding new interests and keeping up old ones. I was taking eleven subjects. I was playing sport—the one school sport I could play, because it was non-contact: badminton. I was involved in a lunchtime debating club. I got the lead role in a play put on by my drama group for our fellow First Years. I was still making *Fush* monthlies. Two of my BSP friends had gone into First Year in Andrew's with me, and I found knowing people already was a big help when it came to making new friends. I could become friends with the people my friends became friends with. Though I may have found it difficult to stay awake on occasion, I enjoyed secondary school.

But there were many things about Andrew's that took a bit of getting used to—for example, the new teaching methods. In History class, I was made to howl like a wolf (best not to ask why). Our Science teacher used to use animal skulls as puppets. Once, he held up a sheep's skull, moved its jaws, and said, 'Num num, I'd taste good with mint sauce!'

My first period of second-level English also provided quite a shock to the system. Coming from the inclusive environment of the Bray School Project, I was used to chatty, friendly, encouraging teachers who were, well, nice. My Junior Cycle English teacher, Mr Agnew, once boasted that no one had ever accused him of being 'nice'.

This man's way of indicating that he wanted the lights turned on was to point at the ceiling. If the noise level in his classroom was irritating him, he would tap his desk ever so lightly with the tip of his pen, until his students were quiet. If a pupil closed his or her ring-binder with an audible click, Mr Agnew's response would be to stop talking and apparently struggle to regain his train of thought. He would then say, calmly but menacingly, 'No clicking.'

On our first day, Mr Agnew came into the classroom holding a coffee mug in one hand, and carrying a plastic bag from Book Stop in the other. He was wearing a light green tweed jacket. We didn't know it then, but the tweed jacket and the Book Stop bag were two things which we would soon come to think of as metonyms for Mr Agnew. Mr A was a portly man. He had a half-ring of grey hair which wrapped its way around the back of his head, from one ear to the other.

The beyond-middle-aged educator moved behind his desk. The class fell silent as he lowered himself into his black, high-backed leather chair. The Book Stop bag stayed on the floor. The coffee mug was placed on the desk.

Mr Agnew cast a disdainful glance around the room. Then he began to speak. 'What is your name?' 'Where did you go to primary school?' In turn, we would all be asked these questions.

The first subject of Mr A's interrogation was the first girl on his right in the front row. He put the 'school' question to her before the 'name' one.

The girl replied that she had gone to primary school in England.

Mr Agnew shook his head, and repeated his query.

'England,' came the response a second time.

Mr Agnew turned to the boy directly opposite him, and inquired in his mild Northern Irish accent, using a deliberate, droll tone, 'What did she forget?'

The boy had obviously attended a better-disciplined primary school than the rest of us. 'England, sir,' he answered.

Mr Agnew nodded slowly, letting out the smallest of evil smiles.

You could almost hear each member of my class shaking in his or her shoes!

I went home that day cracking 'Yes, sir. No, sir. Three bags full, sir' jokes in front of my friends that I would never have dared utter in front of Mr Agnew.

When I arrived at our house, I recounted the events of the school day to my mum, and Mai became furious. Despite my begging her not to embarrass me, she insisted on making a complaint about Mr Agnew's behaviour.

Mai phoned the St Andrew's Headmaster and, using words like 'bullying', 'intimidation', and 'unacceptable', she conveyed her dislike of this English teacher's 1900s-style attitude to education. Our Headmaster assured my mother, however, that Mr Agnew only treated First Years in the manner he did because he wanted our minds to be focused on the important work of his class, and not on extraneous frivolities. Once we became familiar with Mr A's ways, we would no longer see him as a tyrant; we'd recognise that he was, in fact, a teaching genius. Our Headmaster also made the seemingly incredible statement that, by Fifth Year, students were very disappointed if they were not included in Mr Agnew's class.

Remarkably, I grew to appreciate this statement. Mr Agnew only taught me up until my Junior Cert exams. By the time I entered the Senior Cycle, he had retired from teaching. And I and other members of my year found this to be a tremendous shame, because his critical expertise and encyclopaedic knowledge of English would certainly have proved useful for us during Fifth and Sixth Year.

Once we matured a little, we even began to savour Mr A's dry-as-a-desert humour. His classes often took the form more of sermons than of lessons. He'd meander off on the most random of anecdotes, but would always come back to make a central point—either about our English course, or about human existence in general. I remember, one day, he was telling us about a painting which depicted a woman knitting, or something like that, and was entitled 'The Golden Age', or something similar. Mr Agnew explained that a squall of controversy had surrounded this painting, as the artist appeared to be suggesting that the era in which women did nothing except sit at home and knit was a 'golden age'. That wry smile twitched on our teacher's lips, as he opined, 'And, of course, the painting was terrible, because, as we all know, women should be out playing rugby and driving tanks.'

Nothing if not brutally honest, Mr Agnew always let you know precisely what he thought of the work you did for his class. And if he happened to plough through your self-esteem while he was giving you his opinion, well, that was just unfortunate (or maybe not so unfortunate, from his point of view). I was good at English, so I was thankfully not often the butt of his unwelcomely frank comments on students' work.

In class, Mr Agnew would frequently ask pupils to read their essays aloud, so the rest of us could critique their efforts. Being picked to provide analysis always made us squirm. Mr A obviously wanted to sharpen our critical skills, but being forced to tell a classmate what Mr Agnew wanted you to say about the classmate's essay (which was invariably something bad) naturally led to uncomfortable situations.

I was selected to perform this 'critiquing' duty regularly. At a St Andrew's social evening sometime during my third year at the school, my parents approached and introduced themselves to Mr Agnew (yes, including my mum!). He shook their hands and, laughing heartily (a change from the wry smile), he told them, 'Whenever I have something really bad to say about somebody's essay, I call on Ben to do it for me.' I think that was a compliment.

Mr Agnew's standards kept my schoolmates and me on our toes. Those standards gave me an eye for language, an eye that I never would have possessed otherwise. On our first day as members of his class, he told my fellow students and me, 'You're in show-business.' What he meant was that, before creative writing is anything else, it has to be entertaining. After all, if one isn't moving or amusing one's reader, what's the point?

So, in the end, I was thankful for this inimitable man's teachings — certainly a lot more than I thought I would be on that First Day, when I was a 'bullied' and 'intimidated' First Year, dealing with a trip back to the 1900s.

My first year as a pupil at St Andrew's College drew to a close in early June 1998. The end of our last exam was met with predictable 'School's out for Summer!' jubilance, and my friends and I removed all the books and other things from our lockers, stuffed these books and other things into our bags, then sauntered down to Booterstown DART Station together.

On the train on the way home, as we passed Dalkey Station and headed for Killiney, I did what I always did at this point in the journey — I stared out the window. On so many DART trips during First Year, I'd been stunned by the beauty of everything about the view between these two stations. There was this wide arch of a cliff that looked out onto the ocean. In the distance, the sea and the sky blurred together at the horizon. Occasionally, there'd be ships speckled on the water's stillness. Always, the white surf would be tossing itself against the brown rocks, and lapping over and back from the grey strand. On some mornings and evenings, I'd seen the clouds above the waves crack apart, and the yellow fingers of the sun reach down to touch the waves and give the sea a magical shimmer.

As I stared at the beauty, I thought about the previous few months. In May, exactly a year after its founding, I had ended the Nottwel Club. It broke my heart to have to disband my magazine-creating clique. But there were only two or three people other than me who were interested in contributing to the mag, and I wasn't able to continue doing the vast majority of the work. I was too tired, and school stuff was keeping me too busy. As I gazed out the window, I wondered if the free time of summer would allow me to start a new writing project.

That June 1998 day on the DART, I was sitting across from one of my BSP-and-then-Andrew's pals who had been there when the Nottwel Club was born. His voice now pulled me out of my seascape-induced daydream.

'What're you doing tomorrow?' he asked.

'Hospital appointment,' I said.

My checkups in Our Lady's were still fairly frequent: once a month, at least. They were a part of my routine; going to hospital was as normal as going to school. But this particular checkup was an important one. It was my last medical assessment before I went on my first trip away from home without my parents.

The destination for this milestone trip was somewhere I was already familiar with — the Aran Islands. I was going to Irish College, the Gaeltacht — that infamous place to which parents send their children to learn and to speak the Irish language. And of all the Irish Colleges they could have sent me to, Mai and Des had chosen to ship me off to the one on Inishmore: Coláiste Ó Direáin.

Three of my BSP pals came with me to Coláiste Ó Direáin in June '98. We departed for Aran from a hotel in Dublin, with a busload of other Gaeltacht-bound teenagers. My friends and I didn't really know what we were heading into, but we knew we wouldn't see home again for three weeks — that was the length of the Coláiste Ó Direáin course.

I remember getting off the boat in Kilronan, dragging a massive bag of clothes and snack bars and oxymethalone. Teachers from the Irish College were directing us toward the minibuses that would take us to our *teach*s — the houses where we'd be sleeping and eating during our stay on the island.

The fact that this was my first trip away without Mai or Des was a liberating one, and, in that respect, I enjoyed my Gaeltacht stay. Some other aspects of the trip, however, joined forces to create one of those situations where, when you look back years later, you see a worthwhile 'character building' experience, but while you're actually living through the experience, it's akin to a kind of Hell on Earth.

The Irish College regime itself wasn't too bad. We would rise in the morning, gobble breakfast, and then stroll up to the college building for three hours of classes. After these lessons, we'd all return to our respective *teach*s for dinner. After dinner, we'd go back to the college for two hours of sports. In the evenings, after tea in our *teach*s, we all danced ourselves silly at céilis up at the college.

These céilis were often fun — and always nerve-wracking. On some evenings, it would be the turn of the girls to pick which boys they'd like to dance with. On other evenings, it would be the boys who had the choice.

At the close of each Gaeltacht day, after the céili, there was the ritual patriotic rendition of the National Anthem, for which my fellow Irish College students and I used to stand upright and fix our gazes forward. In Coláiste Ó Direáin, however, there was a disagreement between two of our teachers over whether we should sing the traditional words to the anthem, or whether we should sing a 'new age' version, which replaced the term '*fianna fáil*' (soldiers of destiny) with '*laochra fáil*' (warriors of destiny). The teacher who advocated the use of '*laochra fáil*' felt it was a more appropriate term, given the party-political intimations of '*fianna fáil*'. We never knew which version of the anthem we were supposed to sing, until we saw which teacher was going to be leading us in song.

Every night, after the céili and the anthem-rendition, I'd go home tired, ready for the sleep I hoped getting into bed would bring.

But, as I said, it wasn't the Irish College routine itself that I found hard. What I found cripplingly difficult, was being around other teenagers.

With people I didn't know, I was quiet, I was shy. It was hard for me to get to know new people on my own. What happened at Coláiste Ó Direáin was that my BSP pals formed new friendships and relationships, and I didn't.

I remember, during our morning classes, we used to have a midmorning break, during which we'd all head out to a concrete basketball court around the back of the college building. While my BSP companions wandered off and chatted with their newfound mates, I'd stand up against a wall somewhere and try to blend in with the paint.

I also found myself on the sidelines in the afternoons, when all the other Irish College students would be playing sports. I couldn't take part in any game that might result in me getting cut or bruised.

In the final week of that June '98 trip to Inishmore, though, I had a remarkable reversal of fortune — something made me feel very much a part of the Irish College community. During that week, the members of each *teach* had to create a short play in Irish, and perform it for the members of all the other *teach*s. Most groups just came up with sketches that made fun of the teachers. The other members of my *teach* and I had elements of teacher-slagging in our little production, too — along with parodies of TV adverts, and the like. In our production, I played a newsreader, as well as some other minor parts, and the whole thing came with the thrill and the fun I'd always got from the stage.

After my *teach*'s performance, so many people approached me, and told me that I was a great actor, that they'd loved my characters.

On our last day at Coláiste Ó Direáin, we all filled one another's copybooks with notes to remember one another by. And, as I packed my bag to go home, my copybook was as full as anyone else's, thanks to what I'd done onstage.

So, come the end, I was both glad and sad to be leaving Inishmore at the close of June 1998. On the morning of our exodus, minibuses collected all us just-graduated Gaeltacht students from our *teach*s, and brought us and our humungous bags of clothes and other luggage to Kilronan.

I remember standing on the grey pier in Kilronan that morning, waiting to board the Rossaveal ferry. I looked to my right, and gazed at the sandy strand, flecked with brown and green seaweed, where Emma had told me thirteen months earlier that she just wanted to be my friend.

But the view was making my heart break all over again. So I turned to someone who wanted me to sign his Coláiste Ó Direáin workbook. And I thought about how nice it would be to get home.

Before my life as a St Andrew's College pupil began, before I even went to buy books for exciting new subjects like Technical Graphics and Classical Studies, in the early days of August 1997, I held a party at my house.

It wasn't on the scale of the one I'd hosted in June '97. It was a small gathering, for members of my dear Nottwel Club.

I recall ringing up my friends and asking them to come to the party. And there's one call in particular that I remember.

I phoned Emma and Michelle's house, and Michelle answered.

She said, 'Hello?'

I said, 'Hi, it's Ben.'

She said, 'Who?'

I said, 'It's . . . Ben . . . Ben Murnane.'

She said, 'I'm sorry, you must have the wrong number.'

And she hung up.

Convinced it was all a dreadful mistake, I redialed the twins' home number, and once again Michelle picked up.

She said, 'Hello?'

I made sure to stress my syllables. 'Hi. It's Ben From Your Bray School Project Class.'

Michelle laughed. 'Oh, Ben! Was that you just there? I didn't know, you sounded weird, like an American or something.'

Obviously, either my voice or Michelle's memory was having a bad day!

But when I told her about the party, she replied that she and Emma would love to come.

And the two girls did show up, along with most other members of the NW Club. And we all had a good night, crunching on tortilla chips and sipping soft drinks, while sharing our anticipation of entering secondary school.

Yet, it was a strange night for me, too. It was the first time I'd seen Emma since the final day of Sixth Class; and it was odd to be in her company and realise that what she asked for on that Aran beach had actually, at last, come to pass. Emma and I were now just friends, and that's the way we would remain into the future.

After the Nottwel members left my house, I could be found pacing up and down the floor of my bedroom.

I was wondering when they were going to end. These maddening thoughts I was having about Emma.

For a curious, dreamlike period after our conversation on Inishmore, it'd almost seemed as if Emma and I wanted the same thing from one another. But in reality, our positions had been decided on that dull, mizzly evening, with the soft crashing of the sea and the playful antics of our classmates surrounding us — Emma, pleading for my friendship, and me, wandering off on my own, distressed, longing for something I couldn't have.

The upset which hit her as we split from each other to attend different secondary schools and lead quite separate lives was immediate, and temporary; the pain which distilled through me on account of our parting would be slow, drip-dropping into my soul for years to come.

Being in love is not the same as truly loving someone, of course. The two often go hand in hand, are sometimes indistinguishable; though not always. True love dreams of selflessness, of wanting only what's best for the object of its affections. Being in love is one of the most selfish human urges — it's all about what the person you desire does for you.

I'd like to think I truly loved Emma. I wanted her happiness more than my own. But I also needed her, in that most self-centred of ways. And I was utterly obsessed with her.

My obsession was not a daily agony, nor even an hourly pest; it was a minute-by-minute, second-by-second siege of my thoughts. Memories and possibilities to do with Emma flashed through my head constantly, occupying part of my thought process no matter what I was doing. It was a situation so extreme, that if I stopped thinking about Emma for a few seconds, I would be amazed, and say to myself inwardly, 'Gosh, I didn't think about Emma for a few seconds!'

When secondary school began, Emma and I were friends who didn't get to see or even talk to each other that often. So every couple of months, one of us would write a letter to the other. Our letters would contain news and well-wishes — the things friends usually fill their letters with.

As it became clear to me that my love for Emma wasn't going to recede any time soon, I wondered about using these missives as a way of letting Emma know how I felt — just as I had written her that fateful letter, passed to her via a pal, during Sixth Class.

I wrote several 'tell all' missives to Emma in early 1998, but posted none of them.

In the end, my own desperation told me it was better to have a sliver of Emma's friendship than risk not having her in my life at all.

You may consider my obsession incredible; believe me, I did too. And I considered it overwhelming, on evenings after school when I sat on my bed crying; and on nights when I lay awake in that same bed, too empty of tears to cry at all.

Throughout my first year in St Andrew's, and heading into my second, I didn't reveal my obsession with Emma to anyone. Mentors and friends alike didn't know of my heart's secret. And I was lucky, in a way. Perhaps it was the actor in me, but I'd always been quite good at keeping my inner life separate from my outward conduct.

I was particularly careful during that time to hide my desire from my parents. Telling them would have been like letting loose some beast in our house, ensuring that home life was never normal again. There would have been awkward questions, strange silences, and glances of slightly bemused sympathy — none of which I wanted to endure. And yet, I'm sure there were occasions when my frustration over the Emma situation spilled into whatever else I was doing, leading to unexplained outbursts on my part. These outbursts must have left my parents bewildered, knowing that there was some underlying pain in me they couldn't reach.

As I've said, I didn't often meet up with Emma in those days. The first time I saw her in 1998, in fact, was during August, when she and Michelle arrived at my house to star in a short film I'd written. Some of my other friends were going to star in the project, too.

This wasn't my first attempt at making my own movie. I mentioned before that, when I was a kid, I loved superheroes. I even invented an imaginary life for myself, in which I was a superhero living in a cave inside the Sugarloaf. My favourite superhero, though, was the original and best—Superman. In 1995, at the age of ten, I wrote the script for my own Superman movie, 'Superman and Supergirl'. My dad filmed the short film on his camcorder early in the summer of '95.

I played the Man of Steel in my homegrown movie. Immersing myself in the part, I wore blue tracksuit bottoms, and I put on my mum's red knickers over these. I also wore a blue polo-neck with an orange and yellow 'S' taped to it. A red towel was tied around my neck to act as a cape. My sister Ruth, in a similarly makeshift costume, took the role of Supergirl. And I coerced a few of my mates into playing the other parts, including that of the uniquely named villain, 'Super Evil Man'.

My friends were suitably harassed on the day we filmed 'Superman and Supergirl'. They viewed the whole thing as a bit of a laugh, but I saw myself as a brow-furrowingly serious director. I chastised my cast for giggling in the middle of takes. I yelled at them for not treating the project with the respect it deserved. Eventually, after I had criticised everyone into submission, my dad managed to get all twenty minutes of our mini-movie on tape.

A few days later, I was looking forward to seeing the results of our hard work, when Des came to me with a smile on his face.

It wasn't a happy smile. It was a guilty smile.

'Now, Ben, don't get upset,' he said. 'I accidentally recorded over your Superman thing with your sisters' ballet.'

I felt as though someone had flung a full keg of beer, and it had hit me, squarely, in the stomach.

And so my directorial ambitions were put on hold until August 1998.

The idea I had this time was to do my own fan episode of the sitcom *Father Ted*. In the weeks prior to my pals coming to Kilmac to shoot the short film, I beavered away on a script. My anaemically

weak storyline involved two priest-detesting sisters arriving at Fr
Ted's home on Craggy Island, with the intent of murdering him.

We had a lot of fun that afternoon, my friends and I, recording the
short film. Members of my cast even made their own on-camera
changes to the script, in order to give the dialogue I'd written at least
a patina of humour!

But as I said, that was the first time in 1998 that I saw Emma. And,
being the devious, lovesick young man that I was, I invited Emma
and Michelle over to my house for earlier in the day than I invited
the rest of the cast, so I could spend a little while with the object of
my desire and her twin, before we began filming.

And I noticed on that warm afternoon how much Emma had
grown up in just a year. She had become a flawlessly attractive young
woman. Her white face was framed by glowing, shoulder-length
golden-brown hair; her body was svelte and her legs were long. She'd
grown up, but she was still the same Emma, the same laughing and
caring and intelligent girl who had cracked through my shell more
than a year before. To me, just being around her was like touching
the world's deepest magic.

When she departed my house that evening, with my other friends,
once our *Father Ted* 'episode' had been shot, I was a boy shattered.

The unrequited love I felt really was like a drug addiction. Being
in Emma's presence gave me a shocking high. But, once I left her, a
depressive haze would descend on my head. During waking hours,
I'd struggle to find the will to do anything. And at night, I wouldn't
have nightmares, but instead dream dreams of the life with Emma
that was so out of reach. And then I'd hate reality more.

Throughout those periods after meeting up with Emma, I'd feel
despairingly alone.

And it would always be weeks before the hurt, the longing, the
loneliness settled to a bearable level.

After the filming of 'Ben's *Father Ted* Extraordinaire', the remaining
days of 1998's summer holidays trundled by. It wasn't long before I
was back at St Andrew's College, this time as a Second Year.

And September brought with it a brand new subject. 1998/99 was
the pilot school year for Civic, Social and Political Education (CSPE) —
a subject intended to instil in us impressionable teenagers a sense of

social responsibility. Most of my schoolmates considered this new class to be laughably easy, a weekly waste of forty minutes. I, however, thought it was very important for us to learn such things as: When you light a barbecue in your garden, you infringe your neighbour's right not to have smoke blowing over his or her property.

In October of Second Year, my schoolmates and I were treated to a Sex Education seminar. Our year's six forms were split into The Boys and The Girls, and then we were divided into further groups.

So, there I was, seated in room twenty-four of St Andrew's College with around two dozen other teenage lads, still humming with my feelings for Emma, and hoping that somebody was going to say something which made sense to me.

I probably would have been better off looking for a two-year-old to fly to China on his own and bring me back a piece of the Great Wall.

The woman conducting the session spent a good portion of the time raving about how 'hot' her own son was.

She fed us lies — for example, 'All penises are the same size when erect.'

We started talking about homosexuality, and the Session Conductor informed us that gay people are lovely. 'Some of my best friends are gay men.'

A few minutes later, we were discussing acceptable ways of getting sexual pleasure. The Session Conductor told us that she had no problem with oral sex. 'But anal sex is disgusting.' She went to the whiteboard and drew a picture of a cylindrical-looking thing with bits of gunk coming out of it.

'This is a waste pipe,' she told us. 'And that's what the anus is — a waste pipe. Why would you want to stick your precious organ up a waste pipe?'

Somehow, my friends and I managed to survive the assault on logic and human decency of our October '98 Sex Ed seminar, and we continued to endure the everyday school mundanities of study and nagging teachers unfazed.

And yet something inside me just would not die down. Every minute of every hour of every day, I went on missing Emma.

As 1999 began, my heart was still full of these feelings; it was like a balloon on the verge of bursting. I started to think that if I could just share the secret with someone, the pressure might be lessened.

But who could I talk to? I definitely didn't want to reveal anything to my parents. I didn't want to speak to any of my friends about Emma, either. I didn't think they'd understand.

In school at this time, our English classes were not being taken by Mr Agnew, but by a temporary teacher. She was a blonde, bubbly young woman from the United States, possessing that often-inspiring-but-on-occasion-nauseating American enthusiasm for life and everything in it.

One Monday in April 1999, this new English teacher gave us a homework assignment: keep a diary each night for seven days.

I scribbled about different things in my journal on different evenings—a mate's birthday bash, the simple joys of arriving home after an exhausting morning and afternoon in school.

On the Saturday of that week, I was supposed to go to the cinema in Bray with Emma, Michelle, and another mutual female friend. Michelle was sick, however, and so only Emma and our other friend turned up.

I recall sitting on a low wall opposite the cinema on that dazzlingly sunny afternoon, waiting for Emma and her companion. I sat on the wall for over half an hour, until my friends finally appeared. They were very late. I saw Emma striding around the corner, the sunlight tangling itself in her straight hair, and I felt my body become weak and energised at the same time. I leapt up from the wall.

We'd missed the start of the movie, but this didn't seem to matter to Emma. We went ahead and did what I normally would never do—we wandered into the film mid-way through its showing.

The movie we part-saw was *A Bug's Life*. When the end credits started scrolling up the screen, the three of us strolled outside to the heat of the day once again.

We didn't really talk much as we ambled down the Bray street—just haltingly exchanged news. Emma and I hardly ever saw each other, but every time we did, the amount we had to say seemed to dwindle. I was no longer confident speaking to Emma at all—the way I felt about her had made me so scared of Saying The Wrong Thing. I thought carefully about any words I used before releasing them through my mouth.

[59]

Emma, our friend, and I walked through Bray until we reached the DART station. There, Emma and our other pal met with more friends of theirs. The two girls gave me casual farewell hugs, and then I moseyed off by myself. I reached a bus stop and waited for the Kilmacanogue bus.

Seeing Emma on that sunny Saturday caused all my acutest longing to float right back to the surface. But you still couldn't have stopped me from going to that cinema, even if you were offering me all the Michael Jackson merchandise in Neverland.

When I got home, I sat at my desk in my room, and opened up the journal I was keeping for English.

Suddenly, all my most guarded emotions came gushing out of me, spilling through my pen onto the white paper. I spent eight pages explaining my unrequited love for Emma to my temporary English teacher.

We handed up our diary assignments in class the following Monday, and I did not regret submitting mine. It was such a relief to know that someone was going to read about my emotions and discover how I felt.

I was, however, dreading getting my assignment back.

A few days later, my journal was returned to me. I opened it up and turned to the final page, so I could read whatever comments my temporary English teacher had written.

'Isn't it strange how something as beautiful as love can also be so devastating?' she wrote.

7. Expectations

Since my diagnosis with FA in 1994, my parents had searched for panaceas in several places other than Crumlin Hospital.

One Saturday afternoon in the opening quarter of 1996, for example, Mai, Des, Ruth, Jess, and I travelled to see a cheerful old lady, a 'natural healer' who had been recommended to Mai and Des by a friend.

We all traipsed into this lady's house, and she led us into her sitting room. She then performed a test on me in which she pushed down my arm while asking me to resist as best I could. I fought hard, but she was still able to push down my limb with gentle ease.

The healer said she could help me. She gave my parents a bottle of yellow-green liquid, and told them I was to be given a dose of this stuff every day.

The other members of my family were then subjected to the 'arm-pushing-down' test. And apparently there were plenty of things wrong with them, too.

By the time we left the natural healer's house that afternoon, all five of us had been provided with unsightly herbal concoctions in glass bottles.

I never took my medicine, though.

This was Fifth Class, and I was still under the influence of prednisolone. I remember how utter fury filled me that Saturday afternoon. Was this what my life had come to—visiting witches in the middle of nowhere?

It wasn't only because I was angry that I refused to even sample the yellow-green liquid. I didn't know how many calories were in each dose of the stuff. Was this 'medicine' going to make me pile on the pounds?

We never returned to that old lady.

About a half-year previously, I'd visited an allergy specialist. She'd told my parents that I should stop eating wheat.

After this specialist's recommendation, Mai and Des filled up our kitchen with corn bread, corn pasta, homemade pizzas with corn-flour bases. For months and months, all the food I ate had to be wheat free, by order of the parental overlords.

Eventually, however, Mai and Des realised that my wheat-free diet was not doing anything to improve my health, and they let me go back to stuffing myself with the wheat-filled foods that I loved.

I didn't miss wheat too much during my time off it—I was on prednisolone, so, as far as I was concerned, the fewer foods I was allowed to eat, the better. But once I was taken off the steroid, I started wanting to sink my teeth into French breads and takeaway pizzas again, and it was nice to be permitted to do so.

I didn't hold the fact that my parents had prevented me from eating my favourite foods against them. Well, maybe just a little. But I knew Mum and Dad were willing to try anything, if they thought it might improve my condition even slightly. They searched everywhere they could think of for an alternative way of helping me. But they found nothing.

Since my diagnosis, Fanconi anaemia was something that had affected us in bursts, and then it had become simply a pill I had to take every morning, a hospital appointment I had to keep every month. Between the end of Fifth Class and the start of my third year of secondary school, my health stayed pretty much static. I couldn't play contact sports. My energy was low because my blood counts were low. And I tended to get head colds more often than my classmates, because my immune system was weak. The biggest health 'crisis' I had was my skin problem of First Year; but as I experimented with different creams, my dry skin eased.

These were the only health issues I had to deal with between Fifth Class and Third Year. Apart from them, I was well. I was just a teenager whose life was a little different from his friends'.

By now, I'd learned enough about my illness to know that this state of relative wellness wouldn't last forever. The future was not something that scared me, though. I'd no reason to believe that things were going to change any time soon.

When Third Year began, I was feeling determined. The summer of 1999 had been one of strange discoveries for me.

In July '99, my mum's dad died. He was eighty-two, and he had been in a nursing home, his health deteriorating, for several years. But no matter how expected his death might have been, it was still shocking. I remember the day the news came; it was the first time I ever saw my dad cry. Naturally, my mum's tears flowed freely too.

Granda's funeral was held in the church in his hometown of Edenderry, Co. Offaly, and it was beautiful — if one can describe something so sad as beautiful. Moving songs were sung, and moist eulogies were spoken. Through the words and the presence of all those there, I got to know a man I'd never really known while he was alive. Granda had suffered a stroke before I was born. He lived with partial paralysis and a severe speech impediment ever after. Ruth, Jess, and I used to watch him smile as others conversed around him; we used to place kisses on his stubbly cheek when saying goodbye. But this was the most interaction we ever had with him.

Granda's was the first funeral I'd been to of someone close to me. And even though he had been very old, and I was still very young, it was impossible not to think thoughts of my own mortality, as I kneeled in an Edenderry pew, my hands clasped and my head bowed.

We went to the graveyard, and watched the coffin being lowered into the ground. It was an odd feeling — all of us living people, observing the final journey of a dead man. Not so long ago, only the years between fourteen and eighty-two, and the distance between Kilmacanogue and Edenderry, had separated my granddad and me. Now he was an unreachable distance away, and he would be, forever.

There could not have been much more of a radical difference between the feelings July '99 brought for my family, and the feelings August '99 brought. In that latter month, we departed the Emerald Isle for California. We were going to stay with my godfather, Kevin Hayes, and his wife and three children, for three weeks. We spent the first week of our holiday around San Francisco, and the second in LA. During the third week, we rented a cottage in Coffee Creek, in the beautiful wooded mountains of the Trinity Alps, about three hundred miles north of San Fran. Kevin and his family rented an adjacent cottage.

The days slipped lazily by in those California hills. The sun was as bright and as warm as you'd expect it to be, lighting up the loosely packed trees and the smooth tarmac tracks running between them.

There was no television in our cabin, so it was possible at least for a few days to escape the addictive tide of instant news and push-button entertainment. We ate barbecued food, went for strolls in the woods, and chatted to our American neighbours — a middle-aged couple who collected postcards from around the world.

Many an afternoon up in Coffee Creek was spent at a place near our cabin — a place dubbed the 'Man Hole'. As might be suggested by the name, this was a postcard-perfect watering hole at the bottom of some small cliffs, in a clearing amidst all the trees.

I recall sitting there one afternoon, by the side of the trickling river, while my sisters and Kevin's three kids took turns diving from the rocks into the pool of glass-clear water. I wasn't joining them; I hadn't swum in years. I'd taken lessons before I was diagnosed with FA, but once my Broviac was put in, I hadn't been allowed to swim. Even after the catheter was removed, I never got back into the activity.

Sitting by the side of that watering hole in August '99, I remembered the swimming lessons I'd taken at a pool in Dublin before my diagnosis. After each lesson, my mum used to make me shower without my togs on in one of those communal showers — in the girls' dressing room! I wasn't the only boy in the girls' dressing room; we were very young, and our mums wouldn't have been able to come into the boys' changing room with us. I was, however, the only boy who was made to shower naked in front of everyone. Apparently I wouldn't have been washed properly if my togs had stayed on — which is fair enough, but still, I was the only person who had to do it.

I'd also taken swimming lessons at a pool nearer to home, in Bray. That had been traumatic for other reasons. The instructor used to threaten to make us do the backstroke naked if we didn't meet his standards. He also used to threaten to make us stand outside in the cold, naked. Obviously, he had a lot of issues!

I was able to smile a little, ensconced on the green grass at the Man Hole, as I thought about these things.

But then I considered why I had never taken up swimming again, after my Broviac was removed. There had been nothing to stop me from doing so — in fact, the exercise would probably have been really good for me: non-contact, using all those muscles, etc.

I suppose I was scared. Not so much of the swimming itself; I'd enjoyed being in the pool as a kid — the feeling of weightlessness, the warmth of the water against your skin. I just didn't want to be almost-naked around a bunch of other people again. Having FA had made me more conscious of my body. Being poked with needles; having a tube coming out of my chest for three years; becoming obsessed with my weight for nearly a year; having my skin flake apart and being teased about it . . . all these things had made me more conscious of my body.

I'd wanted to touch, to hold Emma so much when were going out in Sixth Class. But I was frightened. I didn't know if my sick body deserved to be held, to be touched; and I didn't know if that sick body deserved to touch someone else's body. That's why Emma had always had to be the one to initiate things — our slow-dance, our kiss . . .

I was glad I wasn't swimming with my sisters and Kevin's children. I would have loved to be that carefree, to have been carefree enough to actually enjoy the kind of thing the other kids were doing. But the truth was, I'd have died of embarrassment before I'd stripped down, put on a pair of togs, and dived into that water.

So, I sat on the bank with the adults, observing while the five younger kids splashed away.

And I was happy. In that moment, I felt a surge of appreciation. Here I was, sitting amidst incredible natural beauty, watching people I cared about enjoy themselves. It was peaceful. I'd been thinking about my fears; but I didn't feel constrained by them. I felt like I could go anywhere from here.

A month before, I'd been mindful of my own mortality. Now I was struck by the terrifying responsibility of actually being alive in this world, and having to meet my own expectations.

And a chance for expectations to be met — academically, at any rate — was hurtling towards me. That's why I entered Third Year determined: the end of that academic year would bring with it my Junior Certificate examinations, and I wanted to make sure I did the best I could in them. For me, 'wanting to make sure I did the best I could' often meant becoming restless with worry.

But the end of '99's summer holidays brought with it another kind of worry, as well. As the new school term was about to begin, my parents received a phone call from Dr Aengus O'Marcaigh at Crumlin

Hospital. Dr O'Marcaigh had replaced Fin Breatnach as my consultant in 1997, after returning from eight years of work and study in the United States. Aengus was a paediatric haematologist; Fin was a paediatric oncologist. Aengus, in fact, had been one of only two paediatric haematologists in the country, when he arrived back in Ireland in '97.

On that phone call in August '99, Dr O'Marcaigh told my parents that he did not think we would be able to rely on the oxymethalone to prop up my blood counts for much longer. The results of my latest blood test suggested that the drug's influence over my counts was waning.

I wasn't sure what to do with this news. I'd been relatively well for so long, I still couldn't see this changing.

But, as August moved into September, I did notice my body weakening.

One weekend afternoon early in September, I was supposed to be heading out for a game of tennis with my dad. I was sitting on the toilet before heading out, when I fainted. I woke up some thirty seconds later on the white-tiled floor of the bathroom, with my trousers around my ankles, and a circle of blood under my head.

My mind beating with the pain of the fall, I pulled up my trousers, attempted to wash my hands, and then struggled into the kitchen. When my mum saw me approaching, scarlet streaks dribbling down my face, she thought that I was playing some kind of prank — that I had spread jam on my face or something.

The tennis match had to be abandoned.

Even after that incident, however, my worsening health was not something I was prepared to think about, as long as I was able to get up every weekday morning and make my way to school.

Third Year required a lot more work than First or Second. I became a stressed-out wreck in anticipation of my first set of State exams.

Mai and Des thought I was taking the whole thing way too seriously. My mum even rang my form teacher, and asked her to have a chat with me about the exams — Mai thought that maybe my form teacher could calm me down.

One morning in the early months of 2000, my form teacher and I passed each other in a St Andrew's corridor, and she stopped me and took me aside. The flood of blue-jumpered students continued to stream by, splitting into tributaries running toward different 'house areas' and classrooms.

My form teacher said to me as everyone else went past, 'You know, Ben, the stuff I say about how everybody should take the exams more seriously, and study more, that's not aimed at you.'

I laughed, told her I knew that, and urged her not to pay attention to whatever exaggerations my parents were feeding her.

Truthfully, though, worry and overwork were wearing me down. I didn't want to see my friends because I felt I needed to study instead. I was even stealing sleep time to use it for study.

Once school was over, we still had two weeks or so before the start of the Junior Cert. I decided that, in order to finely hone my exam technique, I'd need to be somewhere more conducive to sombre study than my own hectic household. I left Kilmacanogue for Clonmel, Co. Tipperary. It was here that my aunt Bernadette, or 'Bing', as she was nicknamed in my family, lived.

I remember travelling down to Clonmel with my dad, in his car. My mind was in near meltdown with nerves. I knew that this three-hour car ride was robbing me of valuable study time. I had to remind myself that there was a reason I was going on this trip: once I got to Clonmel, I'd be able to work myself to exhaustion. Bing's house was the perfect place to do excessive amounts of study, free from parental interference. She was a teacher who lived by herself. Her house was quiet, and she always left me to my own devices.

I said goodbye to Clonmel just a few days before my first Junior Cert paper. As I was leaving, Bing handed me a bag containing four wrapped packages. She told me that this was a present for my exams. I looked at the objects sealed in brown paper; they were all the same size and shape, and each one had a label on it, declaring when the package was to be opened. One package had 'Open Before The First Exam' written on it. Another had 'Open After The First Exam' written on it. The third package was labelled 'Open After The Last Exam', and the fourth 'Open On Results Day'.

As per these instructions, I unwrapped the first package on the night before my first exam. Inside was a lovely clear drinking glass with the word 'Arse' carved into it in graceful lettering. Bing had written a short note to accompany the glass, and this was curled inside the drinking vessel. The note read: 'I know you feel like cursing, but don't worry, the worst part is nearly over!'

And, indeed, the worst part — that is, getting through the first paper — was nearly over. I went to bed after unwrapping Bing's gift, knowing that only a single night lay between me and my first exam, English Paper 1.

7.00 a.m.: I was awake. 7.30: I was leaving the house. 8.20: My friends and I were getting jittery as we sat on the DART. 9.15: I went into the main hall in Andrew's, where the exams were being held.

I took my seat, looked up, and gazed as an invigilator sliced open the sealed bags containing our exam papers.

The paper I had been scared of for what at this point seemed like most of my life was placed in front of me.

And then: 'You may begin!'

When I got home that evening, I unwrapped the second of Bing's packages. The parcel contained another lovely clear drinking vessel. This one, however, had the word 'Feck' cut into it. I unfurled the note Bing had left lying inside the glass. 'I know the end seems a long way off, but the rest of them will fly by!'

Once again, Bing was right. My fortnight of Junior Cert exams flew by faster than I could list all my exam subjects. And once the 'JC' was over, it was remarkable how quickly I adjusted from a state of complete stress to a state of summer relaxation. I felt like a reservoir being refilled. I found myself looking forward to Fourth Year, Transition Year. I knew it would provide a welcome change from the previous three.

After my last exam, I went home to get changed — some friends and I were heading out for dinner. There was one thing I had to do, however, before I got ready to go out.

I opened the bag in which two of Bing's wrapped packages remained. I reached in, pulled out the package marked 'Open After The Last Exam', and ripped off its brown paper. The third glass had the word 'Drink' engraved on it. And Bing's note read: 'Let the celebrations begin!'

Shortly after the end of my Junior Cert, I went into Crumlin Hospital for an ultrasound scan. Since my diagnosis, I'd had ultrasounds relatively regularly to check on the condition of my liver. Oxymethalone was known to interfere sometimes with that particular organ, and this was one reason why it was important to keep an eye on it. Since fainting on the toilet nine months earlier, I hadn't really thought about oxymethalone, or the fact that the steroid seemed to be losing its power over my blood counts. Surely, if there was a real problem, I would have been taken off the drug by now?

I remember having the ultrasound that day in summer 2000. It was a surreal experience — and not for any medical reason. I was in the x-ray wing of Our Lady's, lying on my back in the darkened ultrasound room. My sweatshirt and t-shirt had been pulled up, so that my tummy was exposed; sheets of blue tissue paper were tucked under my t-shirt and under my trousers at my stomach.

The ultrasonographer, the specialised radiographer conducting the scan, was sitting beside me. In front of her was a monitor, and in her hand was an object somewhat like a computer mouse, a 'transducer'. When the ultrasonographer rolled this transducer across my stomach, images of my insides would appear on the monitor.

The ultrasonographer looked down at me. She squirted some bluish jelly onto the transducer, and rolled the thing around on my tummy, spreading the jelly all over my belly.

'You have wonderful abdominal muscles,' she remarked. 'Do you swim?'

'Not since I was a kid,' I replied.

'Do you play a lot of sports?'

'No,' I said.

'With a stomach like that — don't tell me you're a couch potato!'

I left the x-ray wing that day with a smile on my face, and a few days later, I wandered happily into Crumlin Hospital again — this time for a bone marrow aspiration.

Since my first visit to St John's Ward in the run-up to Christmas '93, I'd had my bone marrow aspirated every year. So, this test was not one I was worried about either.

Besides, by now, I was definitely enjoying the anaesthetics they'd give me when I had the aspirations. There was some kind of curious pleasure in letting all my worries drift into the ether as I surrendered to the drugs.

When I groggily awoke after each aspiration, I was always in the recovery room beside the operating theatre. After a while, I'd be wheeled down to whichever bed was mine for the day in St John's.

Once I got to my St John's bed, I knew the numbness would begin to fade, and my hip would start to hurt like hell. An irritating wooziness would descend, lasting for hours.

But for those few moments before they wheeled me away, lying on my back in the recovery room, with the beeping and whirring of medical equipment in my ears, my surroundings still felt as though they were a product of my dreams.

I mentioned earlier that many of my childhood holidays were spent in Connemara, Co. Galway. My parents rented a cottage there almost every summer when I was growing up. While we were in Connemara, Mai, Des, Ruth, Jess, and I would go for exhausting mountain walks, laze around on the perfect beaches, and even take boat trips out to Inishbofin island.

It's strange, sometimes, the things you remember most from your childhood. I recall one occasion, when I was around eight, standing on the yellow sand of Glassillaun Beach in Connemara. A wealth of shells was dotted about me. Translucent purple jellyfish were washed up on the shore in front, and behind them, the gorgeous blue of the tide was rocking back and forth like a slow metronome. To my left, dark rocks hosted rock pools teeming with tiny creatures. Beyond the rocks, hidden in distant mists, was the grey outline of Inishbofin. To my right, the hulking mass of Mweelrea, the highest mountain in Connemara, loomed.

My feet were planted on the strand, and I was beside my dad, who was holding the string of my precious navy and green kite. The kite was sailing high above us, rippling with the wind.

Des asked me if I would like to hold the kite. Excited, I said I would.

But as he passed it to me, the white string slipped out of my small hands. And my beautiful kite breezed away, flying until it was only a diamond-shaped dot on the horizon . . . and then not there at all.

Tears formed on the rims of my eyes. I blinked, and these tears slid down my cheeks.

My dad smiled, and urged me not to worry. We'd buy a better kite, he said. And he brightened my mood with images of my kite reaching America. I giggled as I thought of it floating past the Statue of Liberty, and sailing above the Manhattan streets.

But I still felt crushed by what had happened. I'd watched as something dear to me slipped away — slipped away because I didn't grip tight enough.

But the reason I'm bringing up Connemara again is that, in 1996, my parents bought a cottage there. Our new 'home from home' was in an area called Shanaveagh, a couple of miles from the famous Kylemore Abbey. Shanaveagh was located between Renvyle and the oddly named Currywongaun. Our nearest shop was a mile and a half away, in Tullycross.

It was a nice house. The views were amazing. All around our cottage, knobbly mountains curved and spiked; hills poked from the ground like the shoulders of buried giants. From our kitchen, you could even see the smooth surface of the sea — in the distance, mirror-like water wandered into a little inlet.

Streaming through the right-of-way leading up to our house was a narrow and shallow river. The river meandered around the back of our cottage, and thick bushes hung over it on either side. When we first got the cottage, I spent many a day in my blue wellies, splashing through the shallow water winding behind our house, pretending I was some kind of Jurassic explorer (wherever there were a lot of bushes, I liked to imagine there were dinosaurs hidden in them).

I didn't always have to play by myself. Sometimes, friends of mine would come down to Shanaveagh with me and my family. There weren't many things of interest to kids or teenagers out in the wilds of Connemara, however. So, you could only bring each friend down to the cottage once. No pal would be gullible enough to come with you and put up with all that boredom a second time.

I enjoyed my times in Shanaveagh, though. And the slower pace of life there was something I grew to savour more as I got older.

In July 2000, after my Junior Cert and my June checkup in Crumlin, my dad and I were down in the Connemara cottage. My mum and sisters were still up in Wicklow — they were planning to join us in a few days' time.

One afternoon, Des and I were both reading in our Shanaveagh living room, when the sharp rings of the telephone cut through the quiet. It was my mum on the line. She'd been talking to Dr O'Marcaigh.

Aengus had told Mai that my recent ultrasound scan had revealed growths on my liver. While these were not cancerous, he believed they'd been caused by my years of using oxymethalone. This, combined with the fact that the steroid was losing its power to improve my counts anyway, had led Dr O'Marcaigh to conclude that I should be weaned off oxymethalone, starting immediately. After six and a half years, I was to stop swallowing those tiny white tablets in the mornings.

My relationship with oxymethalone had mostly been a sweet one — without it, I would never have lived. But there had been bitterness, too. It had led to my awful acne, and it had made me bloated.

There'd even been confusion in my relationship with oxymethalone. On occasion, the steroid had set me ahead of my peers. During Fourth Class, my voice broke before any of my male classmates. When I joined the school choir, I was asked to mouth the words to the songs rather than sing them, because my voice was so much deeper than everyone else's!

These were the things I thought about, when Des told me that I was going to be weaned off oxymethalone. I was able to reminisce to myself — this seemed like good news. I wouldn't have to remember to take my pill anymore.

'What happens now?' I asked my dad.

I wasn't prepared for the answer to that question.

Des said that Aengus hoped a bone marrow donor could be found for me very soon.

And then I remembered that the oxymethalone had been the only thing keeping me alive. Once it was gone, I could be dead within a few months.

All of a sudden, I was terrified. And furious. I didn't understand why this was happening. I yelled at Des.

'This is your fucking fault!' I shouted. 'Your fucking deformed genes!'

I went into my room and banged the door. I screamed.

Then I fell down onto my bed.

I just didn't understand why this was happening.

8. Onstage

There is a word for a rapid reversal of fortune— 'peripeteia'; I've seen it used to describe moments in plays when the expectations of characters are suddenly turned on their heads. I could hardly think of a better word to describe the way the course of my life reversed, following that July afternoon in Connemara.

Some months earlier, during the Easter holidays of 2000—after my mock Junior Cert exams, but before the real deal—my parents, my sisters, and I had gone to Paris for a short, relaxing break. We stayed in a friend's apartment, a cosy place in the southeast of the city. My pal Michael—the guy whose dad took Mai and Des up Mont Blanc—was camping in southern France at the time. He took a train up to Paris to spend a few days with us.

On one of those days, Michael and I were in the apartment, sitting at a table by a window in the living area. The window was open, and sunlight was gushing down on top of us. A light breeze was making the white curtains ripple. Below us, people walked this way and that, on the grey pavement of a Paris side street.

Michael and I were bored. We were searching for something to entertain us.

'Are you ever going to start doing the magazine again?' Michael asked me. It was a question he'd asked before. In fact, since the demise of the Nottwel Club in 1998, several of my friends had wondered if there would at some point be another mag.

I was beginning to think that producing the magazine would be a great thing to return to. After all, Fourth Year was going to be easier than the Junior Cert years; I would again have the time to put together the issues. Besides, I missed my magazine. I missed having my own personal outlet for my writing, for sharing my interests with my friends.

'Why not?' I replied. 'Let's start now!'

For the rest of that afternoon, Michael and I worked on the first edition of a new series of magazines. Michael sketched an image for the cover of the zine, and I began writing some articles. Our new mag was christened *Totally Fushed*—another Terry O'Driscoll term. And even though the Nottwel Club was long dead, I made 'Nottwel' the 'company' that published *TF*.

Totally Fushed: Special Edition (#0) was completed in the days following the end of our Junior Cert. The mag had the headline 'Nottwel™'s Back For The Post Jr Cert Hangover!' on the front, under Michael's picture.

My dad drove me to his office one weekend, and I photocopied the mag while he waited. I took the copies home, sorted them out, and stapled each of them. I posted copies of *TF* to some pals, and gave other friends theirs by hand. I gave copies to BSP friends and Andrew's friends—whoever I thought might be interested.

Everyone appeared to be delighted that Nottwel was back.

I was delighted, too.

Which is one reason why it was so crushing to discover, on that July afternoon in Connemara, that my health issues were all flying back into focus. I was supposed to be going into Transition Year, supposed to be finally getting some freedom to pursue the things I was interested in. I didn't feel ready to fight for my life.

Shortly after returning from my family's Connemara cottage in July 2000, I sat with Dr Aengus O'Marcaigh in a consultancy room in St John's Ward of Our Lady's Hospital for Sick Children.

In one corner of the room there was a blue leather patient's couch, suspended above which was a curtain. This curtain could be pulled in front of the examination couch, whenever privacy was required. At either end of the consultancy room there were filing cabinets, stuffed to the brim with patients' charts.

Aengus had my chart on the desk in front of him; the tall, thin, pale doctor searched for a particular page, while I waited. This was my second chart; the first had become so full that the Crumlin team couldn't cram anything more into it. Aengus read out my latest blood results. He sombrely informed me that, because I could no longer rely on oxymethalone, I would need to start coming into Crumlin every few weeks, for regular blood transfusions.

'You could survive for a year, maybe longer, on transfusions,' he said. 'After that . . .'

Aengus told me it was up to me whether or not I had a bone marrow transplant. Half of those FA patients who underwent matched unrelated BMTs did not survive. But a transplant offered at least a chance of survival. Without a BMT, I probably wouldn't live longer than two years.

It didn't seem like the kind of decision I should have to make at fifteen.

'There is something else we can try,' my consultant continued, 'though it's not guaranteed to work.'

Aengus proposed that I inject myself with erythropoietin (EPO) for a trial period of a few months. You may have heard of EPO before — the overseers of the cycling profession have been trying to rid their sport of the substance for years. EPO is a hormone that stimulates the production of red blood cells, boosting the oxygen-carrying capacity of the blood. In other words, it increases haemoglobin levels. In the case of cyclists, it can help them ride faster and for longer. In my case, there was a possibility that EPO would keep my energy above the 'critically low' point, at least while we waited for a transplant donor to be found.

I tried to take in everything Aengus was saying to me. I'd spent so many years being relatively healthy, it was impossible to accept that this period had vanished forever. Now, it was as if I were standing before a giant locked door. I was holding the key in my hand, but above the door was a colossal neon sign, flashing the words: 'WARNING! IF YOU ENTER YOU MAY DIE WITHIN A FEW MONTHS! BUT IF YOU DON'T ENTER YOU WILL DIE WITHIN TWO YEARS!'

EPO wasn't a 'cure'; only a successful transplant could stop my bone marrow from failing, once and for all. I knew that I'd have to take a chance on a bone marrow transplant someday. But delaying that day from arriving for as long as possible seemed like a good idea to me. Maybe the EPO could give me a new normality, a normality like the one oxymethalone had given me.

'I'll try the EPO,' I said to Aengus.

My doctor nodded. 'I know,' he said, 'that this whole situation is ...' he seemed to be struggling, as if about to say something he wasn't used to saying, '. . . a bollocks.'

I was shocked. Since I'd first met him three years before, Aengus had always been polite and calm. His use of the curse word was completely out of character. I laughed when I thought about it afterwards.

But, because it was so out of character, it touched me. It made me feel as though Aengus weren't my doctor anymore; he was my ally, fighting with me, down in the trenches.

We left the consultancy room, and Aengus took me to a nurse. I watched as she showed me how to inject myself with EPO.

The nurse's demonstration was conducted on an orange. She held a needle poised on a syringe in her gloved hands, showed me the correct angle, and then pushed the needle into the orange.

'Got it?' the nurse asked, withdrawing the needle from the round fruit.

I nodded numbly. I was about to become some kind of junkie, sticking needles into himself just to make it from one day to the next.

Thrice a week, I had to give myself shots of erythropoietin. I'd pinch a lump of skin on my stomach, and push the needle straight in. I'd feel cold tingles as the pink fluid flowed into me.

The EPO did not bring up my haemoglobin level immediately. Even though I was injecting myself with the hormone, I was still 'transfusion dependent'. Once a month, I had to go to St John's Ward and have a cannula inserted. Then I would sit for four hours while two bags of O+ blood trickled into me.

Usually when I went to get my transfusions, I'd be coming from school—Mai or Des would pick me up and bring me to Our Lady's. I used to sit on a hospital bed, or in a hospital chair, with textbooks and copybooks in front of me, trying to complete the school day on my own. No matter how often I did it, though, I never got used to doing schoolwork in hospital. There were too many distractions— from bald kids wheeling up and down the corridors on plastic tricycles, to the ever-on TVs, to just the fact that there was so much sickness around me. What I preferred to do was my own writing.

'I look over at the door opposite me,' I wrote one day while having a transfusion, 'a symbol of free air beyond; unlike the trapped, sterilised place where I write. Danny, a massive blob of nine-year-old Kerryness in the bed beside me, asks if I like school. Normally I'd say no; right now, I'm thinking yes. I go for the compromise, "Ah, it's not too bad." Any place is better. The medical straps from three machines attached to me are like chains in a prison. The physical pain from the needle in my arm is like a metaphor for a deeper tear in my emotions. Meanwhile, Tracy Chapman whispers in my ear that I can die now, my true love won't come for me. Oh, no. There are those with nothing, but for once can't I be selfish? The ink flowing is like blood. Mine. My life on paper. Someone else's blood flowing into me.'

For months and months, I sat and waited while someone else's blood kept me alive.

Before Transition Year began, I had to tell my friends that I'd been taken off oxymethalone, and that my future was now uncertain.

I remember speaking to one group of pals in a McDonald's restaurant in Bray. There we were with our greasy yellow fries and our dripping brown burgers, and I was revealing this serious news.

I spoke to another few mates as we sat in the Bray Cineplex, waiting for a movie to start.

The reaction of my pals was always similar. Each person stayed silent for a few moments, then offered sympathetic words, or asked a question. I know from experience how difficult it is to be on the receiving end of a friend's bad news. You feel a rush of worry. You don't know what to say, or even if there is anything to say. You want to help, but don't know how you can.

One hot evening late in July, I was outside SuperValu in Greystones, Co. Wicklow when suddenly, purely by coincidence, Michelle sauntered by.

She noticed me, smiled, and said 'Hi!'

I strolled with her along the pavement, and we began catching up with events in each other's lives.

All that stuff about the oxymethalone, the blood transfusions, the bone marrow transplant, and the EPO—I just didn't know how to tell her. I could only use the two words which most summed up how I felt about my life at that point.

'I'm dying,' I said.

There were tears in my eyes, but I refused to let them roll down my cheeks.

'Oh, Ben,' Michelle responded, tossing her arms around me. She told me that Emma was on holiday, but said that she would ask her to call me once she got back.

The following Sunday afternoon, I was on my own in the Kilmacanogue house, doing some work for the latest issue of *Totally*

Fushed on the computer in my parents' room. At around four o'clock, the phone rang.

'Hello?' I said.

Emma was on the other end. Michelle had told her what was happening to me.

'I'm so sorry, Ben,' Emma said.

For as long as I'd known them, Emma and Michelle had been spiritual individuals, devout in their Christian beliefs. Emma told me on that Sunday afternoon, 'You know, in my religion, we believe, you know, that God has decided what's going to happen to everyone, and I just . . . I don't understand why He's doing this to you.'

That phone call was the first time in ages that Emma and I just talked. We talked about her holiday in Florida. We talked about movies. We talked about music. She talked some more about me.

'You've been a really special friend to me, Ben . . . I . . . Everything you've been through, everything you do, your magazine . . . You deserve to be famous . . . I . . . In a way, I look up to you.'

I laughed. 'I'm not sure I'm a good role model!'

'Oh, you are,' she replied.

The love in my heart threatened to spill into my speech.

'Well,' I said, 'I hope you . . . you and Michelle . . . I hope you both know how much you mean to me.'

I heard Emma mumble 'Yes.'

I wanted to say so much more, but I didn't.

After that conversation, though, my friendship with Emma and Michelle grew closer than it had been at any point since Sixth Class. I visited their house several times over the next few months, and they even came to Crumlin with me to meet Aengus.

During the summer of 2000, I went to the 'Festival of Hope' Christian rock concert with the twins. This was held in a marquee in Greystones. At the concert, I received a free Bible and a handbook on being a good Christian. The handbook featured a cartoon character named 'Ben Born Again'.

I remember standing outside that marquee in Greystones while the light of the day faded from the sky; blue became navy, and the green trees became black silhouettes.

'Have you ever let Jesus into your heart personally?' a young woman with an American accent asked me. She offered me a Festival of Hope Commitment Card. On this, I was supposed to write my name, address, and telephone number. There were three boxes on the card, and I was supposed to tick one of them: 'Received Christ', 'Recommitment', or 'Other'.

I glanced down at the card, then looked up at the young American lady. 'Actually,' I said, 'I'm not Christian.'

The woman gave me a look which said, 'Well, what are you doing here?'

It was a fair question.

I thought about the days behind, the days ahead, and the fact that I could sense my own body weakening. But I still didn't feel the pull toward God that Emma and Michelle felt.

Maybe Emma, Michelle, and all those people in the marquee had it right, though. They knew there was a better world beyond this one, a world we could only get to through death. All I could see after this life was a blackness, an end to all thought and feeling; I couldn't even imagine how that would happen — to suddenly just stop.

Once the last band had left the Festival of Hope stage, I went back to Emma and Michelle's house, while I waited for my mum to pick me up.

I sat with the twins in their living room. We were chatting away, when Emma and Michelle's dad came in. He asked me to join him in a room across the hall. I followed him. The twins' dad left the doors to both rooms open; so, from the room I was now in, I could still see Emma and Michelle, sharing sisterly conversation.

The twins' dad turned to me. 'The girls told me about your situation, Ben,' he said. 'That must be pretty shit.'

I let out a slight laugh. 'It's . . . yeah, I guess,' I replied. I didn't know what else to say. I felt the way I'd felt when Aengus told me that my situation was 'a bollocks' — I had allies, I had people by my side.

'Well, if there's anything I can do, or if there's anything any of us can do,' the twins' dad offered.

'No,' I responded. I glanced over at Emma and Michelle, who appeared to be bickering. If the blackness I imagined death to be had an opposite, it was the feeling of warmth I was filled with at that moment. 'Just, obviously, if the girls keep in touch . . .'

A few days after the start of my Transition Year, I was reminded once again of my conversation with Emma on an Aran strand. In September 2000, almost my entire St Andrew's year departed for Inishmore. We were escorted by some teachers, most of them from the Irish department.

This Andrew's Aran trip was like a replay of the BSP one — we stayed for three days and two nights. We even slept in the same Kilronan hostel. On the second day, most of my year went on a bicycle tour of the island. Instead of going on the cycle, two other non-bike-riding students and I went on a walking tour of Inishmore. One of the Irish teachers acted as our guide.

We got to see a lot of the island on that stroll. We trudged through grassy fields while trying to avoid sheep shit; we clambered over wire fences and stepped over low stone walls. The four of us eventually ended up in a pub. Here, our teacher-guide bought (non-alcoholic!) drinks for the other teenagers and me, before we rejoined our classmates as they returned from their cycle.

The day of that island stroll was an odd one for me. All the health worries that had come crashing down around me during the summer were still dangling in front of my eyes. When the two schoolmates who were on this walk with me lagged behind to chat to one another, I found myself pouring my heart out to a St Andrew's Irish teacher I had never spoken to before. I told her everything about my illness: how I was injecting myself with EPO, how the constant blood transfusions were affecting me, how I felt about having a bone marrow transplant, how I could watch myself getting paler and paler as I looked in the mirror every day . . .

The Irish teacher just listened, empathised.

I found it hard to talk to my friends about all the details of my illness. Talking to this adult stranger was so much easier. There was something comforting about the distance between this teacher and me, something comforting about the knowledge that my sharing would have no consequences.

On a Wednesday morning shortly after we returned from the Aran trip, all six forms in my year lined up alphabetically in the main hall of St Andrew's College. My classmates and I had been waiting for this day since the middle of June. Finally, it had arrived. The nervous anticipation was as thick as margarine.

Each Transition Year student was handed a sealed A5-size manila envelope containing his or her Junior Certificate results.

I didn't want to open mine in front of my friends. My schoolmates were still hugging each other, grinning and slapping each other's backs, when I left the main hall. I briskly walked to one of the boys' toilets, went into a cubicle, and locked the door behind me.

I ripped open my brown envelope and scanned my list of subjects and my grades.

Eight As and two Bs.

My first feeling was relief — it was a relief not to be disappointed! The happiness came next, splashing inside me like playful water.

After I returned to Kilmac and showed my results to my parents, I went into my room, and opened the last of the packages that Bing had handed me before my first Junior Cert exam.

Inside was, of course, a fourth transparent drinking glass. Written in slender, misted lettering on this glass was the word 'Girls'. Bing's accompanying note read: 'Now it's time for the real celebrations!'

By the middle of September 2000, Fourth Year was in full swing. And, even though I was still getting sicker, I was enjoying school. We got to sample a host of new, non-exam-based subjects. The core subjects of English, Irish, Maths, and a European language (in my case, German) were still compulsory, but even the atmosphere in these classes was more relaxed. I remember, one day, sitting in class at the start of a Maths lesson. Our teacher came into the room, and a bunch of students in the back row held up a banner which read: 'Mathematics Is The Science Of Avoiding Sex With Women'. Our teacher was on form with his retort, too. 'How come you are all so good at it, then?' he asked.

Among the new subjects I was taking were Psychology, Media Studies, and Politics. I especially liked Politics. One of the things we had to do for that class was collect three newspaper articles every week. Each week, we also had to write an opinion piece on one of the articles.

On 4 October 2000, a story which appeared on the front page of *The Irish Times* struck very close to home. The piece, by Dick

TWO IN A MILLION

Ahlstrom, informed readers that, in the United States, a couple had 'used genetic selection of their embryos to have a baby whose cells could be harvested in an effort to save the life of their seriously-ill first child'. The 'seriously-ill first child' was Molly Nash, a girl with Fanconi anaemia, or, as *The Irish Times* mistakenly called it, 'Franconi anaemia'. Molly's brother, Adam, was a 'test-tube baby', born after being genetically screened as an embryo. He was chosen for life by Molly's parents over their other embryos because his cells were the best match for a transplant for Molly. Adam was born on 29 August 2000. On 26 September, stem cells from his umbilical cord were transplanted into Molly. The chances of the girl surviving FA were now much, much higher.

The procedure which led to the saving of Molly's life, however, had conservatives and 'pro-lifers' up in arms. They were appalled by the idea of embryos being genetically screened, and they were outraged that the Nashs' unused embryos had been simply discarded. According to them, the latter was tantamount to murder. A spokesperson for the anti-abortion group Life was quoted in Ahlstrom's article. 'That kind of screening belongs in the farmyard,' the spokesperson said.

It was fascinating to have the disease I was suffering from placed at the centre of the world's news. Naturally, my Politics opinion piece that week was on the Molly and Adam Nash saga. Our Politics teacher, however, brought the divisive 'genetic screening' topic up for discussion in class himself, before he had collected our homework. When it came to my turn to speak, I mentioned that the illness I had was the same as Molly Nash's. Our teacher looked embarrassed. He then spoke to me after the lesson, saying he hoped he hadn't put me in an awkward position by raising the subject for debate.

It was a strange experience, listening to the opinions of my classmates. Several students said they could never support the kind of embryo screening that had taken place in the Nash case. I knew that there were two sides to the issue, and that to some people it was immoral both to mess with the natural birth process and to destroy embryos which could become fully grown human beings. But it was hard to see how this side of the argument had any merit, when I was locked in a real-life battle with the illness that had almost killed Molly Nash. I didn't say it in class, but I felt as though these students were making personal statements against me, against my right to exist. I wasn't Molly Nash, but she had the same disorder as me; this procedure could potentially be used to save the lives of many more people with my disease. Any word spoken against it felt like a dismissal of my life.

Every Friday afternoon during Transition Year, normal classes were suspended. That's because Friday was the day we went on Outward Bound trips. Our year was split into several Outward Bound groups. Every week, each group did a different activity—climbing, canoeing, hill walking.

I couldn't take part in most of the Outward Bound sessions. But I wanted to be involved as much as I could. So I insisted on attempting the hill walk.

On the afternoon of the trek, my classmates, two teachers, and I travelled by minibus up into the Dublin Mountains. When we arrived at our destination forest, we hopped out of the bus, and began to walk through the woods at a steady pace.

After a while, we started to follow a rocky path uphill. I fell behind. I saw yellow spots in front of my eyes; the trees and sky swirled into each other . . .

I called out to one of the teachers to stop. He paused and turned around. The other teacher went on ahead with the rest of the group.

I sat on a tree stump by the side of the mountain path, feeling as though all my energy had rolled back down the hill. I opened the black and blue rucksack I had with me, and took a drink from the bottle of water I'd brought.

After some minutes, I felt ready to go on. The teacher and I climbed to the top of the hill, where everyone else was waiting.

I knew they had waited because of me, and I fought to hold back tears. All my life I had tried never to fall behind. I had certainly never wished to slow anyone else down. I felt crushingly inadequate.

I didn't go on any more Outward Bound trips.

There were other, after-school, activities that I did get involved in, though. I joined the Model European Parliament; I was on a debating team which took part in a competition in Bray.

I remember we had to write our own speeches for the Bray debate. When I got up to speak, I had the entire text of mine on pink flashcards. I don't think that's really the point of flashcards, but it didn't matter — I'd memorised what I'd written. During my speech, a middle-aged woman with short blond hair let out a snort of derisive laughter at one of the arguments I was making. For a moment, I felt a rush of anger. I wanted to shout, 'Do you know what I'm fucking going through just to be able to stand here? Unless you need someone else's blood to keep you alive, unless you're prodding yourself with needles every second day, unless you know what it's like to know that you could be dead in two years — SHUT THE FUCK UP!' But I didn't say any of that. I went on with my speech.

Another activity our teachers encouraged us to take part in early in Transition Year was Gaisce — the President's Award. In order to receive this accolade, a young person aged fifteen to twenty-five must complete four separate challenges. The four areas of challenge were Community Involvement, Physical Recreation, Personal Skill, and Adventure.

At first, I didn't like the idea of doing Gaisce. But when my friends signed up, it seemed silly to leave myself out.

For my Gaisce Community Involvement, I worked for an hour a week in the Bray School Project. I remember the first afternoon I went to help in BSP. I stood in the main corridor of the school, waiting to speak to one of the teachers. Framed photos of past BSP Sixth Classes were hung on the walls, and I spotted a frame labelled 'Class of 1997'. Within this one frame there were around thirty photographs — one for every member of my old class. I remembered the day these pictures were taken — a bright, hot day toward the end of our time in the school. The photos had supposedly been arranged in random order, but Emma's picture was placed next to mine. There we were, our beaming twelve-year-old faces immortalised side by side. I couldn't help but smile.

For my Gaisce Physical Recreation, I played badminton, the school sport I'd kept up since First Year. Of course, I had to take it easy during those badminton sessions. I didn't want to end up seeing yellow spots and almost fainting. Thankfully, there were always far more players in the Andrew's sports hall than there were courts for us to play on. Usually, as much time was spent sitting against the wall waiting for a court as actually on one.

The Personal Skill I put down on my Gaisce form was acting.

Upon leaving First Year, there was one thing that made me distraught. I'd been part of an after-school drama class run by Mr Malachi Friel. But Mr Friel only provided lessons for First and Fourth Years. So, after First Year, I'd had to give up this great class. When Transition Year began, I was finally able to return to Mr Friel's drama group.

Between First and Fourth Year, I obviously had to look elsewhere for my acting fix. During Second Year, for a pair of terms, I attended the Gaiety School of Acting's Young Gaiety Saturday course. Unfortunately, however, we didn't do a whole lot of actual acting in the Young Gaiety. What we did do, was play 'drama games'. For example, pretending we were lampposts, and being told to walk as lampposts would walk if they could; or, pretending we were lemons in glasses, and being told to walk as lemons in glasses would walk if they could; or, pretending we were trees, and being told to walk . . . well, you get the idea! Exhausted from all this imaginative walking, I chose not to return to the Young Gaiety for a third term. I withdrew from acting cold turkey.

The withdrawal symptoms I suffered during Third Year really made me realise how much I loved the stage. I began to look upon it as the only place where I felt truly at home. On the stage was where all my pain fell away. I felt safe there; it was much easier to interact with other human beings through the lines of a pre-learned script than it was to interact with them in the randomness of the real world. Onstage, I was alive in my lines, making a character myself; I was in command of my surroundings. I fed on the audience's energy and its expectations. And, sometimes, while I was acting, there were these moments of perfect intensity, when it was almost as if something beyond me were feeding my performance. Those moments supplied a buzz worth pursuing again and again.

In November 2000, after one of his drama sessions, Mr Friel asked me if I would audition for the play he was going to direct for the St Andrew's One-Act Drama Festival. The 'One-Act' was held in Andrew's every February; schools from all over Ireland could compete, and the festival adjudicators were always accomplished theatre people. 2001 was to be the One-Act's thirteenth year.

The play Mr Friel was planning to direct for the 'home team' was *Sorry, Wrong Number*, a thriller by Lucille Fletcher, set in 1940s New York. The play's story involves an invalid woman who, while trying to phone her husband, accidentally overhears a conversation between two men who are plotting to murder someone. The rest of the play focuses on her attempts to stop the killers before it's too late.

That November, I auditioned for *Sorry, Wrong Number*, and landed the part of Sergeant Duffy. Duffy is the bumbling and uninterested policeman whom Mrs Stevenson, the invalid woman, phones to alert of the forthcoming murder. He dismisses Mrs Stevenson as a crank. Duffy appears in just two scenes in *Wrong Number*, so my total time onstage was going to add up to only about seven of the play's twenty-five minutes. But I still had the second largest part in the production. The part of Mrs Stevenson was given to a Fifth Year girl named Belinda.

Sorry, Wrong Number had a cast of fourteen. We all rehearsed hard in the months leading up to the One-Act. A lot of the work, particularly during the final few weeks, was done at weekends.

Finally, the date of our performance arrived — Tuesday 13 February, 2001: opening night of the One-Act. Ours was the second play on Tuesday, which meant our curtain went up at around a quarter past eight.

On the day of our production, I stayed in St Andrew's after lessons ended. I went to the library and tried to get stuck into some homework, but I was too giddy to get anything done. After a while, I met my parents and sisters for dinner in a nearby Italian restaurant. Mai, Des, Ruth, and Jess would all be attending the night's performance, of course.

At around half past six, I left the restaurant and headed back to Andrew's. As I entered the school grounds, I looked up. Hanging above the gates was a banner announcing the One-Act Festival.

I went into the school building through the main entrance, passing a duo of students who were getting ready to sell tickets for the night's plays.

'Are you nervous?' one of them asked me.

I smiled. 'No,' I replied, not entirely truthfully. There were butterflies flitting in my stomach, but I saw that as a good thing. The nervous energy would push me forward. I'd never become terrified before a performance; I never got stage fright. The stage was the one place where I couldn't be frightened.

I walked the length of the school, and arrived at my locker. I took off my navy uniform jumper and my blue and white tie, and put them in the locker. Then I did something of astounding stupidity, the reason for which is still not clear to me.

During my first scene in *Sorry*, I was supposed to be given a bag containing my lunch. It was vital that I be handed my lunch, and appear to be eating onstage, because the whole idea of the scene was that Sergeant Duffy was more interested in his food than in Mrs Stevenson's trying to alert him of an impending murder.

For use in the 'lunch' scene, I had brought with me to St Andrew's that morning a brown paper bag containing a tuna sandwich, an apple, and a Danish pastry.

I now took this brown bag out of my locker, and placed it on the floor beside my locker. I guess maybe I thought it'd be easier to grab the bag in a hurry if I didn't have to open my locker first.

Anyway, after I had put the bag on the floor, I went off to the classroom that the cast of our play was using as a dressing room. I threw on my costume, and one of my female co-stars applied my makeup and put talcum powder in my hair, to make me look older.

At about 7.45 p.m., the first show of the thirteenth One-Act Drama Festival—a production of Tom Stoppard's *Shakespeare* by Holy Child School—got underway. As my schoolmates and I were next up, it was almost time for us to get into position backstage.

I went to my locker to grab the brown paper bag.

The bag wasn't there.

Fuck.

I panicked.

What the fuck was I going to do?

I tried to calm myself. I had to think logically. The bag did look like rubbish—maybe it'd been picked up and dumped by one of the cleaning staff.

I looked in some of the bins in the area around my locker. But all the old rubbish sacks had been removed from these bins, and new ones put in.

Now I was terrified.

What happens if I don't find the fucking thing?

I sprinted up the school corridor toward the main hall and the stage.

What the fuck am I going to tell Mr Friel and everyone else?

As I ran, I spotted about a dozen rubbish bags piled up under the St Andrew's sports notice boards.

I stopped.

I began pulling at the knots at the tops of the bags. When a knot wouldn't open quickly enough for me, I tore the sack with my hands.

I ripped open about five black sacks, and then . . .

Thank fuck!

There it was.

My brown paper bag was heavily crumpled, but it was clean, and the food inside looked edible.

The waves of fear subsided.

I sped away from the ripped rubbish sacks like they were somebody else's problem. My heart still pounding, I joined the rest of the cast backstage. Then, for the first time since my hair was powdered, I could actually think ahead to my performance.

Once my fellow thespians and I got onstage, our rendition of *Sorry, Wrong Number* went gloriously well. The audience seemed rapt; everyone clapped suitably loudly at the end. After our bows, the other members of the cast and I came off the stage grinning excessively; we congratulated each other with boy-to-boy hugs, girl-to-boy hugs, girl-to-girl hugs, and boy-to-girl cheek kisses!

Following the third and final play of the night—St Columba College's production of John Godber's *Up'n'Under*—the two One-Act Festival adjudicators, one male and one female, stood up to offer their comments on the evening's entertainment. The male judge spoke about our production. He praised my portrayal of Sergeant Duffy, saying that I'd been like a cross between Columbo and Chief Wiggum from *The Simpsons*!

Two nights later, following the concluding productions of the festival, the One-Act awards were being presented. The St Andrew's main hall was far more full of people than it had been on either of the other evenings; all the blue and grey foldout chairs facing the stage were occupied, and people were gathered at the back of the hall, near the doors, as well.

I was sitting with some friends, several rows from the stage, as the judges read out the names of those who'd won Certificates of Merit. *Sorry, Wrong Number* was given two certificates; our sound effects operator received one, and a girl who had played a hospital receptionist received the other.

Next, the Runner-Up Best Actress and Best Actress awards were presented. I applauded loudly as Belinda was given Runner-Up Best Actress for her brilliant performance as Mrs Stevenson.

Then, they got to the Best Actor awards.

'First, the runner-up,' the adjudicator announced. 'Ben Murnane, St Andrew's College, for Sergeant Duffy in *Sorry, Wrong Number*!'

People in the packed hall cheered and clapped. My friends looked at me. I clenched my fists and whispered a thrilled 'Yes!'

I stood up and walked toward the front of the hall, smiling at my parents and sisters as I passed them. I climbed the steps. The St Andrew's Headmaster held out his hand; in his other hand was my award.

I was on the stage, and all my pain was falling away.

9. On the runway

By early 2001, one thing was clear. The erythropoietin was not going to work. I'd been injecting myself with the hormone three times a week for months, but my blood counts had not improved; I was still getting blood transfusions regularly. EPO is a substance that stimulates the production of red blood cells by the bone marrow. But the marrow has to be capable of stimulation for the EPO to be effective. My marrow was beyond repair.

Aengus met with me, to tell me a matching donor had been found in England. He then explained what was involved in a bone marrow transplant.

First, I'd have a new Broviac inserted. Then, I'd have radiotherapy and chemotherapy. Next, I'd get my new bone marrow. Then I'd spend between five weeks and three months in hospital, while we waited to see if my system would accept the donor's marrow. If I survived the transplant, I'd still have to take a year out of school; I'd need to be kept in isolation, at home, so I wouldn't get any infections. Even a simple cold could be life-threatening, to a fragile post-transplant body.

I listened to all this. I knew the risks; I now knew the procedure. But I'd already made up my mind. I couldn't turn around. This was my one chance at more life.

I told Aengus that I was ready for a bone marrow transplant. The Crumlin team started making plans to admit me to St John's. The end of March '01 — that's when the transplant was set to happen.

By now, I was getting infections nearly every month. Usually, these were just debilitating head colds. I might have high temperatures, or feel nauseous. But, however I was feeling, I didn't want to let my health distract me. I still had things to keep me busy — not the least of which was Fourth Year.

One of the things Transition Year is famous for is the work experience programme, which involves teenagers finding themselves jobs for a couple of weeks. Members of my St Andrew's year had to spend ten days, two working weeks, at work. It was recommended that students find two places in which to work, one for each week.

Back in September 2000, a friend of mine had pointed out that *The Irish Times* was running a competition for Transition Years: Write a two-hundred-word piece on anything to do with the media, and, if your article is published, win a week's work experience at the paper.

In October, I penned a short piece about the media's coverage of the Molly and Adam Nash case, poking fun at—among other things—the *Times*'s misspelling of the word 'Fanconi'.

On 22 November 2000, my dad phoned me from his office, to offer congratulations. I asked him what he was talking about. He said that he had *The Irish Times* open in front of him, and he was looking at my article.

It had been published! A national publication had printed something I'd written—and I'd won a week's work experience. I spent the rest of the day grinning.

A woman from the *Times* subsequently got in contact with me about arranging dates for my work experience. We decided on the working week from 26 February to 2 March.

So, at 10.15 a.m. on 26 February, I entered *The Irish Times*'s D'Olier Street offices. I had met another St Andrew's Fourth Year lad on the train on the way into town. This guy was also going to be doing work experience at our nation's 'quality' broadsheet.

Several floors up in the elevator later, we found ourselves in the company of four other students from different schools. Our whole group was instructed to go down to the canteen for free drinks. Down we went.

I remember being glad that someone I knew would be working with me at the newspaper. It was easy to feel out of my depth as I wandered through this strange building, its narrow corridors strewn with half-eaten Chinese takeaways and week-old copies of *The Irish Times*.

When my fellow Fourth Years and I were eventually led out of the canteen, we were taken to a meeting room. We sat against a wall, while the *Times*'s Editor and representatives from the paper's various departments discussed that day's newspaper and their plans for the next day's. It was a fascinating 'fly on the wall' experience. I don't think anyone even acknowledged our presence throughout the entire meeting—so we really were like flies on the wall.

After lunch on that first day at the *Times*, the other Transition Years and I were introduced to Shane, a tall, bald subeditor. Shane took us to the buzzing newsroom. He was a friendly guy, who raved about what a great President he thought Bill Clinton had been. He also let us in on a few *Irish Times* secrets. Shane told us that certain words — for example, 'itinerant' — couldn't be used in the paper, as they might cause offence.

My first day of work ended with Shane showing me and the other Fourth Years *The Irish Times*'s printing press. It was several storeys high, and made a lot of noise. We gawped at the giant rolls of newspaper paper; these were shaped like toilet rolls, but were as tall as humans. We watched as Tuesday's Education and Living supplement was printed. Shane pulled a copy of the supplement off the conveyer belt, and held it in his hands. 'Now that's good quality,' he said, feeling the paper. 'I mean, it's not like a book or anything, but, you know, it's good enough quality.'

The next morning, the *Times* sent my group to the Lindsay Tribunal, or the 'Tribunal of Inquiry into the Infection with HIV and Hepatitis C of Persons with Haemophilia and Related Matters'. I know what a person with haemophilia is, I thought as I went into the room where the tribunal was in session, but what's a person with Related Matters?

This was the last time I felt like making a joke, however, until long after I came out of that room. Inside, a certain consultant was being questioned about accusations former patients and the parents of former patients had made against him. He was an important witness; he was an erstwhile director of the National Haemophilia Treatment Centre, and was considered to be, in the words of RTÉ News, 'the leading doctor treating haemophiliacs through the 1970s and 1980s'.

The last time I'd seen him, it was through the window of my room in St Anne's Ward, as he told my mum that I had a rare blood and bone marrow disorder. It was so odd, now, to see once again the man who diagnosed me with aplastic anaemia, as I continued to struggle with the failing health brought on by Fanconi anaemia. He had told my mum that I might have only six months to live; I was still here, seven years later — and I was still dying, too: my current consultant had given me an outside shot at surviving for another year without a transplant.

On that Tuesday in February 2001, this man was asked why he told a patient whose blood was being tested for HIV that he should go ahead and try to have a baby with his wife. He was asked about an incident during which he allegedly left the room after abruptly telling a couple that their son had HIV. The doctor was asked about a claim that he held a consultation with an AIDS patient's father in the middle of a common corridor.

I just sat there and watched; the whole situation was horrifying. Over two hundred and sixty haemophiliacs had been infected with HIV and hepatitis C, because the Blood Transfusion Service had given them contaminated blood-clotting agents.

I remember when news of the tragedy first broke. My dad's friend Terry—the 'founder' of Nottwel—had been a regular blood donor for years and years. He was such a committed donor, in fact, that he had won the Transfusion Service's highest award, the Porcelain Pelican, which is only given to a donor after his or her hundredth donation. When he heard of the HIV/hep C scandal, Terry lifted his Porcelain Pelican from its place in his home, took it out to the garden, and smashed it against the ground.

Terry had felt furious; I felt scared as I sat in on that day of evidence at the Lindsay Tribunal. I needed other people's blood to stay alive, and one of the results of the Blood Transfusion Service scandal was a decline in the number of people willing to donate that vital, life-giving liquid.

My week's work at *The Irish Times* came to an end after lunch on Friday 2 March. I was given a key ring and a t-shirt, and told I could go home.

I couldn't help but feel a little sad as I left the *Irish Times* building for the last time. My eyes had been opened during my five days there. I'd seen how a newspaper was run and how it was printed; I'd gone to exhibitions, a play, and a press conference; I'd been interviewed by a real journalist; and, I'd encountered a face from my childhood that I thought I would never see again.

My second week's work experience had a lot to live up to.

I spent that second week at our national broadcaster, Radio Telefís Éireann.

On the morning of Monday 5 March, I took the DART to Sydney

Parade Station, and then walked up to the RTÉ complex. It was a thrill just strolling through the gates, just being in the place that all my favourite TV shows were broadcast from. I was star-struck, and I hadn't even seen any stars.

This may sound extremely strange, but I thought of the RTÉ complex as being like a space station. There were huge satellite dishes, and there were windowed walkways connecting some of the buildings. It all looked very space-agey. I daydreamed that I was an intergalactic warrior, here to be debriefed after a successful interstellar mission.

In the letter RTÉ had sent me about my work experience, I was told to ask for Cathy Jaruzel. So, when I got to the right building, I did.

Cathy Jaruzel didn't work there anymore.

The letter had also told me to bring two passport photos with me. The woman behind the reception desk now asked me for my photos. I handed them over.

I waited while an identity card was whipped up for me.

Presently, I was on my way to TV Sport, my assigned department. My contact in TV Sport was to be Mary Banks.

Mary Banks didn't work there anymore.

After a while, another woman came to meet me. As we climbed up a staircase, she politely apologised for the fact that, due to the foot-and-mouth crisis that was gripping the country at the time, not a lot was going on. 'Monday is usually quiet anyway,' she added.

It certainly seemed that way — and not just in Sport. As we passed an empty Current Affairs section, I spotted a sign which read 'Take The Day Off'.

Eventually, I did make it to TV Sport. As there wasn't much to do, however, I was allowed to spend most of the day watching TV or on the Internet. Much of the rest of the week was the same. I watched more daytime TV during those five days than I ever have in a concentrated period before or since.

Still, even all that sitting around was tiring. I left RTÉ after my first day with sore eyes. God, your parents are right when they talk about too much TV ruining your sight, I thought.

But I was wrong. My eyes weren't sore from too much screen-watching.

I had another infection.

By the following morning, my eyes were red and puffy; there was gunk oozing out of them, congealing, and sticking them closed. I had to wear sunglasses in RTÉ, just to hide them.

By the next night, the pain and the oozing had become worse. My mum had to take me to Crumlin. When we got to Our Lady's, we were told to go to the Accident and Emergency at the Royal Victoria Eye and Ear Hospital on Adelaide Road.

Mai and I waited with the vending machines in the Eye and Ear A&E for what seemed like a long time. Eventually, I was seen by the doctor on duty. She prescribed me an antibiotic, and slowly my infection cleared up.

But, for those minutes I spent waiting in the A&E, I was scared. I just wanted to see properly again. I could hardly think with the pain, but the thoughts that did get through were about the transplant. I wished they'd hurry up and give it to me, so I could be free of these infections.

'Open wide, now.'

I did as the dentist asked. I didn't mind visiting the dentist. What I did mind was visiting the dentist in Our Lady's. Even for normal things that everybody else had to do, like getting their teeth checked, I had to go to hospital. The dentist had to report to Dr O'Marcaigh.

'Did you notice this before?' the mouth-doctor asked me.

'What?' I said, as he took his gloved fingers out of my mouth. I didn't know what he was talking about.

'You have a white growth there,' he pointed, 'on the underside of your tongue on the right side. It looks like . . . I don't know what it is.'

Cancer?

'It's probably something we should get checked out,' the dentist concluded.

Horrible possibilities flew in and out of my head. I knew the statistics about FA and cancer. I knew there was a chance that, if I survived the BMT, I would have to face a battle with cancer down the road—I just never thought I'd have to fight cancer before my transplant. Was this what I was now going to have to do? There was a white growth in my mouth. What else could it be?

The Crumlin dentist referred me to the Dublin Dental Hospital.

There, one Dr Stephen Flint took a look at me.

Being inspected by Dr Flint was a little bizarre. The Dublin Dental is a training hospital; so, Dr Flint had a posse of about half a dozen students with him while he was looking at me. I was sitting there with my mouth stretched open, and Dr Flint was fondling my tongue with his latex-gloved fingers. As he was doing this, he described what he was seeing to the students who were standing behind him. The students were huddled together like a bunch of penguins, staring at me.

Dr Flint took some photos of my tongue.

'Well, Ben,' he said, 'I'm concerned that this might be pre-malignant, and I think that's our dilemma, really.'

Pre-malignant. My growth wasn't cancerous yet, but it could become so. And because I was due to have a bone marrow transplant, Dr Flint was in two minds about how to proceed. He called my case 'uncharted territory'; there weren't too many cases like mine 'in the literature'. Should he remove the growth? If he did, my tongue could become dangerously infected. If he didn't, and the growth became cancerous, I could be in an even more serious situation.

'I'll have to discuss this with Dr O'Marcaigh,' Dr Flint said.

I'd promised myself I wouldn't let my health distract me. But, by the middle of spring 2001, it was getting harder and harder to stop it. Everything seemed to be clinging to me at once, like leeches sucking on a body: my tongue growth had to be dealt with; there were the preparations for my transplant; infections were still bothering me. It was hard to concentrate in school. There was Emma and there was my health—these were the two trains of thought which just wouldn't stop.

On one of my afternoon visits to Our Lady's, Dr O'Marcaigh took me into that consultancy room—the one in which we'd discussed putting me on EPO—again. I didn't know what Aengus wanted to speak to me about this time.

But I soon found out.

We were going to talk about depositing sperm.

Of course, because I had FA, my chances of fathering a child were slim to begin with. But once I had my pre-transplant radiotherapy, even those slim chances would vanish forever. If I deposited sperm before my BMT, it could be frozen and possibly used years later in IVF treatment.

Aengus told me that there was only one sperm bank for under-eighteens in the Republic of Ireland. He then started to explain the mechanics of depositing sperm.

'Do you know how it's done?' he asked. 'They give you a beaker and you masturbate until —'

'I know how it's done!' I interrupted.

When I got home that evening, I phoned a friend to see what he thought of the 'depositing sperm' idea.

'I'm not sure I like the notion of going into a cubicle and wanking into a beaker,' I told him.

'It's not as if they're in there with you!' my pal laughed.

'No,' I admitted.

Maybe it was just because I was embarrassed about 'wanking into a beaker'. Or, faced with having to cling for years to hopes and chances, maybe I actually felt safer knowing for certain that I couldn't have children. Maybe I thought no woman would ever want to parent a child with me.

Whatever the reason, I never deposited sperm.

After my eye problem had cleared up, after my two weeks of work experience, by mid-March, Dr Flint and Dr O'Marcaigh had decided that the better option was to remove my tongue growth. So, one sunny day, I went to the Dental Hospital to have part of my tongue cut off. There was now only a fortnight until my transplant was to begin.

I fasted the night before my Dental Hospital procedure. Thanks to my yearly bone marrow aspirations, I was used to being under general anaesthesia. Fasting is required before you're put into a general anaesthetic state, as it ensures that you don't puke up your stomach contents, or suck those stomach contents into your lungs, while you're unconscious. For my tongue-growth-removal procedure, I was going to be given a local, not a general, anaesthetic. But I assumed I still needed to fast.

Mai and Des both came with me to the Dental Hospital. After a while, the white-coated, tall, grey-haired, bespectacled Dr Flint came to see us, to apologise for the delay. He said we'd have time to go off and get something to eat before he was ready for me.

'But Ben's fasting,' my mum pointed out.

Dr Flint looked shocked. He laughed, and told us in his soft English accent that it wasn't necessary for me to be fasting — local anaesthetics were not the same as general ones! He insisted that my parents take me to get some food. After all, when he was done 'butchering' me, I probably wouldn't be able to eat normally for quite a while.

Mai, Des, and I returned to the Dental Hospital after I had stuffed myself full of lasagne and chips. I was taken to the room where Dr Flint would be performing the procedure. I sat in the dentist's chair, and was offered a pair of huge goggles. These would shield my eyes from the light shining onto my face.

Dr Flint arrived, and the action began.

I was asked to open my mouth as wide as I could, and to keep it open. Dr Flint injected anaesthetic into the right side of my tongue. The muscle tingled before turning numb and heavy. Dr Flint sewed stitches through the entire right side of my tongue; he pulled my tongue over to the left side of my mouth, so he would have a clear view of the growth. One of Dr Flint's students held the end of the suture, to stop my tongue from twitching, while the doctor himself sliced away the little white menace. After the white patch was removed, the hole where it had been was sewn up with dissolvable stitches. When the numbness faded, it felt like there was a porcupine living on the right side of my mouth, stabbing me with its spines.

'Just don't eat solid food for a while,' Dr Flint said. 'And take some painkillers if you need to. And hope,' he smiled, 'that it doesn't get infected.'

The week before I was due to be admitted to Crumlin Hospital for my 'matched unrelated donor' bone marrow transplant (or MUD BMT), I underwent a bone marrow harvest. A harvest is similar to an aspiration, but more marrow is extracted. The marrow is then frozen for possible future use. It was a BM harvest that my sister Ruth had years before, after Jess was diagnosed with FA. Ruth's marrow was put 'on ice' in case something happened to her and she wasn't around to give a fresh sample when Jess needed a transplant. My marrow was being extracted for a very different reason. If my MUD transplant went horribly wrong and my body rejected the donor's marrow, my own harvested sample could then be transplanted into me, to return me to my pre-BMT state of health.

The days immediately after my harvest ticked quickly by. And then the last Friday in March arrived. I'd told Aengus weeks before that I was ready for a bone marrow transplant. Now I really had to be ready. The following Tuesday was my date of admission. This day, Friday 30 March, was my final day of school.

After all my classes, I cleared out my locker, packed my books into my bag. As I left St Andrew's, I hugged and said goodbye to my friends. I'd appointed two 'subeditors' to take care of *Totally Fushed* business while I was in hospital. There wouldn't really be that much to take care of, however. Production of new issues had stopped. I just hoped I'd be around to start it up again.

My mum picked me up from Bray DART Station on Friday afternoon and drove me home.

Just as we were coming in the back door, into the kitchen, the phone rang. Mai picked up the receiver.

I climbed the steps that led out of the kitchen, and went to my room. I dropped my schoolbag on the floor, and looked around.

I loved this room. When we moved into our Kilmacanogue home, my room had been grey and empty. Then my parents put colourful clown wallpaper on the walls, and Mickey Mouse curtains over the window. During my first year in secondary school, my cousin Ailbhe, my dad, and I repainted the room. I wanted it to convey a sense of magic and adventure. So we painted the floor sky blue, and added white clouds as well. We painted my ceiling black; we stencilled silver stars onto the blackness, and dotted glow-in-the-dark planets here and there. The curtains in front of my window were now orange, and my four walls were bright green. Each wall had a beautiful mural on it, painted by Ailbhe's skilful hand.

On this Friday evening, my blue and white desk was still cluttered with assorted school notes and under-construction articles for *Totally Fushed*. These were things I would have to return to when I got out of transplant.

There was no 'if'; it was 'when'.

I left my room, and strolled back into the kitchen. I was hungry, and was going to search our fridge for a snack.

Mai was still in the kitchen. She'd just hung up the phone, and there was a worried look on her face. She gazed up at me as I came down the varnished wooden steps.

'That was Aengus,' she began. 'The English donor has backed out. The transplant's been postponed.'

10. Walk

I don't know if I screamed. I probably screamed at Mai. That irrational screaming people do just as a release — it doesn't matter who it's directed at. Then I left the house. I had to walk, just walk, be moving. I couldn't feel myself. I was suspended in some horrific dream. I was too angry to cry. A thousand thoughts entered and left my mind in seconds.

It couldn't be true. How could this happen? After I had prepared, after I had told my friends, after I had stopped working towards my summer exams. Now that I was ready for the biggest challenge of my life, where had it gone? And how long would I have to wait to face it again? How could I build myself up for it again? How could I now return to the life I had cut myself off from?

I came out of our driveway and walked briskly down the lane to the road. I didn't turn toward Kilmacanogue Village — I couldn't be around people. I headed in the direction of Rocky Valley Drive. I was still wearing my school uniform, though I had taken off my tie in the car on the way home. The top two buttons on my shirt were undone. It was a mild spring evening; the sun was poking through the clouds. An easy breeze cooled my skin.

I put my hand into my pocket, looking for a tissue to wipe my nose. My hand hit my mobile phone. I took the phone out. I needed to talk to someone. A friend. Someone who would listen, just listen, and not try to shade the conversation with pleasantries or empty humour.

But who could I call? There had never been any one friend, one person I knew would understand and hear me out no matter what. I'd always had many different friends who appealed to different sides of me. I could talk movies with one group, politics with another. My various groups of friends rarely interacted with each other. I was caught between them, never quite sure what to say about one crowd while I was with another. They were all great friends. The best. I would stand with them through anything, bleed for them. But there was no one I knew could give me the empathy I so selfishly needed in that moment.

Then a name arrived — Emma. Why shouldn't I phone her? There wasn't anyone in the world I thought more highly of. True, we hadn't seen each other that much since Sixth Class. But she'd always been caring, had often sent me cards or letters. And last summer, we had seemed to be growing closer again.

I found the number of Emma and Michelle's house in my phone's phonebook, and pressed 'Call'. It was Emma herself who answered.

'Hello?' she said.

'Hi. Emma?' I still found it hard to tell the difference between her and Michelle's voices over the phone.

'Ben? Hi! How are--'

'Not good. I . . .' I told her that the donor had backed out, that the transplant had been postponed for an indefinite amount of time, that I felt utterly lost, that I didn't know what to think of the world or of myself.

She listened, told me I was strong, and that she was sure everything would be all right.

Then: 'Would you like to talk to Michelle?' she asked.

'Okay,' I replied.

And suddenly, I knew there could be no holding them inside any longer — these feelings that I'd nursed for four years like wild animals in cages. Thoughts came at me like water hurtling from a crumbling dam. I remembered. I remembered the ups and downs since Sixth Class, remembered how this girl's glow had guided me through them all. I remembered how my feelings for her had both tortured me and propelled me forward; how in days of confusion, they had been the one thing I was sure of. What if death was only months away? What if I never got another chance to speak those three precious words?

'I love you, you know,' I said.

'What?'

'I love you.'

Silence.

'I'll get Michelle,' Emma murmured.

I waited for Michelle to pick up the receiver. And walked on, alone.

11. Transition

Weeks passed after that desperate telephone confession. I didn't hear anything from Emma. I felt as if I were stuck on a rock somewhere in the middle of an ocean, screaming and screaming; everything inside me was screaming and screaming — but no one could hear me, there was no one to share things with.

At the most vulnerable moment of my life, I'd told the girl I loved that I loved her. And she'd said nothing.

On my own, at night, when the curtains were drawn and the door was closed, and the glow-in-the-dark planets were peering down at me like eerie cats' eyes, I felt as though my insides were reaching into the blackness, grasping for something that wasn't there.

It hurt so much.

Then, as April became May, Emma replied to one of my text messages. She, Michelle, and I arranged to meet. The three of us met at Bewley's Café on Grafton Street in Dublin, on a bright Saturday afternoon.

When the twins showed up, we said our hellos, and then wandered into the café. The girls ordered coffee. I picked up a scone, then went to get a soft drink.

My nerves had always danced when I was around Emma. But today they were doing the jig of their lives.

I took a paper cup from the top of a stack — I was going to fill the cup with Diet Coke. I was so jittery, however, that I didn't know what I was doing. I placed the cup under the Fanta tap. My cup was half full of orange liquid before I realised my mistake. I cursed myself, but didn't empty out the Fanta. I just filled the rest of the cup with Diet Coke.

The twins and I paid, and we sat down at a table.

'So, how are things?' Emma asked me.

'Fine,' I said.

'And you have a new bone marrow donor now?' Emma continued.

Not long after the English donor's backing out, the Crumlin team had found a willing donor in the US. My BMT was on track again; 20 June was my new admission date.

'Yeah,' I said to Emma.

I no longer cared about the transplant. I probably wouldn't survive it anyway; and if I did, I'd still have to live the same hollow, aching life I was living now.

'Why did the other donor back out?' Emma asked.

I told her we didn't know; for reasons of confidentiality, we weren't allowed to. Because the fresh marrow for an MUD BMT has to be extracted from the donor and then transplanted into the recipient within twenty-four hours, the donor can theoretically back out at any moment up until he is actually put under general anaesthesia to have his marrow harvested.

'And,' Emma went on, 'what are your chances of coming through the transplant with this new donor's marrow?'

'Same as before,' I replied. 'Fifty/fifty.'

'Well,' Emma said, 'then you don't need to worry, Ben. I mean, if there was a less than fifty percent chance you'd survive – if it was sixty/forty or something, then you might be worried but fifty/fifty . . . I'm sure you'll be fine.'

I wanted to shout at Emma. How could she possibly know what it was like to face the fact that you could be dead in three months' time? How could she possibly know what it was like to wake up every morning and barely have enough energy to make it through the day? How could she possibly know what fears haunted me at night?

In that moment, the person I loved more than any other friend or any family member, was also the person I hated most in the world.

My mouth was dry. 'Yeah,' I croaked, in response to Emma's theories.

I didn't want to talk about the transplant anymore.

I reached into my black and blue rucksack, and removed two copies of the newest *Totally Fushed*. 'I brought these for you,' I told Emma and Michelle.

I handed the magazines to the twins, and pointed out a particular feature. I'd reprinted an interview Michelle conducted with Emma in Sixth Class. The interview was on the subject of acting, and it first appeared in *TFM* #2.

The girls giggled as the article brought back buried memories of our Bray School Project days.

I took a sip of my bizarre fizzy orange/diet cola combination, and resisted a reflex to retch. I broke a chunk off my scone, and lifted the chunk towards my mouth.

Nerves made my grip on the chunk too tight. It fell apart in my fingers; crumbs cascaded down my sweatshirt and onto my lap.

Emma and Michelle stared at me.

I wanted to be sucked into the air. To vanish. I wanted to cry. Or scream.

Instead, I laughed.

God, how I needed an arm around my shoulder just then. Or someone's hand to hold.

As the weeks approaching June 2001 started to shrivel into memories, I had to go to Our Lady's Hospital for my pre-transplant assessment. This was a series of tests designed to confirm that I was fit to have the BMT.

I trudged from hospital wing to hospital wing that day, with my parents in tow. I was subjected to sinus and chest x-rays, and an echocardiogram; I was prodded by various experts—an ear, nose, and throat doctor, an ophthalmologist.

One of the tests I had was a pulmonary function test. During this, I was asked to blow into, and to suck air out of, a tube attached to an elaborate machine. The process reminded me of using an inhaler, which I had to do when I was seven years old and asthmatic (my asthma, thankfully, cleared up before I was diagnosed with FA).

The pulmonary function test was performed in a gloriously white, sanitary room. Unfortunately, however, the woman conducting the test seemed to be a bit of a headcase. She kept calling me 'Paul', and insisted that I wasn't blowing into the machine hard enough.

'I'm sure you can do much better than that now, Paul,' she criticised repeatedly, as though I were a three-year-old.

When I got the printout showing the results of my pulmonary function test, I brought it to Dr O'Marcaigh. He said he didn't know why the woman had been telling me to try harder—the results were perfectly normal.

Most of the tests in my pre-BMT battery were held on the same day. There was one, however, which took a day all to itself — my psychological assessment.

The assessment was conducted by Dr Gina MacDonnell, a psychologist at Our Lady's. Gina was a short, slim woman, with reddish hair and a lightly freckled face. She had a voice which went from calming, soft tones to a sort of endearing high pitch when she became excited about something.

The psychological assessment comprised two two-hour sessions, with a break for lunch between them. During the course of our four hours together, Gina gave me various exercises to do, and asked me various questions. The purpose of these exercises and questions was to determine whether or not I was mentally ready for the transplant, and also to determine where my talents and weaknesses lay. The more the Crumlin team knew about me, the better they would able to meet my needs — throughout the transplant and beyond.

The results of my psychological assessment confirmed that I had high literary intelligence. In most other areas of the assessment, however, I scored below what the average person would. This was not because I performed any of the assigned tasks incorrectly, but because I hesitated over them and exceeded the time limit for many.

I remember being pretty pissed off when I received the results. 'The tests were all bullshit anyway,' I said to my parents. After all, any system which told me I was 'slow' had to be a load of crap.

I walked out of the room, leaving my mum clutching my assessment results. As I went, I decided to sum up the psychological profession. 'Freud liked his mother because she was hot,' I announced. 'Simple as that.'

Throughout the months and weeks leading up to June '01, people showed me astonishing kindness. Classmates I'd rarely spoken to offered to help in whatever way they could; family friends did likewise. The teachers in BSP put together a framed collage of photographs from my days at the school, and gave it to me as a 'good luck' gift. The collage included shots taken on the Inishmore trip, as well as a picture of me in a duvet-like woolly jumper, reading a poem about a whale that I wrote in Second Class; there was also a photo of the 1997 BSP Pupils' Council, which I had been elected to.

The goodwill of all these friends, elders, and strangers started to make me think that there were other things for me in this world besides a girl who wasn't in love with me. I began to feel the pressure of the forthcoming transplant again. I stopped not caring. I had family, I had friends, I had talents . . . and I wanted to live.

The days of waiting were difficult. My friends would talk about their summer plans, where they were going on holiday. I had bigger summer plans than any of them, but I didn't want to talk about those plans. I couldn't talk about them. Beyond the broad outline that Aengus had given me, I had no idea what to expect from my bone marrow transplant. The 20th of June was a target I just had to get to. What happened after that was in the hands of my doctors, and in the hands of Luck.

After my pre-BMT assessment, there was really only one big thing standing between me and my transplant: the end of Fourth Year.

In the last week of the St Andrew's summer term, a special 'Transition Year Night' was held. On TY Night, every student was presented with a certificate declaring that he/she had got through Fourth Year. Depending on how well the teaching staff thought you'd performed, your certificate could be labelled either 'Satisfactory', 'Merit', or 'Distinction'.

Other accolades were presented on TY Night as well. Every student who had proven himself or herself fluent in Irish received a gold, circle-shaped badge, or fáinne. Every student who had completed all his or her Gaisce challenges received a President's Award.

While I was given a gold fáinne, I did not get a Gaisce award. I'd completed my Community Involvement, my Physical Recreation, and my Personal Skill challenges, but I couldn't complete my fourth and final Gaisce challenge — the Adventure. This challenge involved going on a two-day walk, cycle, or canoe trip. The only one of these that I could conceivably have done was the walk. Throughout all of Fourth Year, however, I'd been too weak to even attempt such a trek.

It was tough watching my friends march onto the stage to get their Gaisce awards, while I sat in the audience. I should have been up there with them. I would have been, were it not for Fanconi anaemia.

Once the final days of Transition Year passed, there was just a fortnight left before my admission to Crumlin. I decided that it would be nice to fill this fortnight with mad adventures.

So, soon after school ended, I got drunk for the first time in my life.

While staying in a friend's house, I downed two cans of beer, four or five shots of vodka, four or five shots of whiskey, and I stole many swigs from a bottle of cognac. I had great fun falling onto the couch with my eyes closed — 'It's so cool! It's like a rollercoaster!' I'd say to my friends, feeling a little lurch in my stomach as I intentionally fell face-first into the soft cushions.

That night, I stumbled around a lot, knocked over a bowl of olive oil, collapsed into the bushes and had to be hauled out by my buddies . . . It was terrific!

My friends and I spent most of the night in a chalet, away from the main house. I recall walking in circles on the wooden floor of the chalet, spilling my feelings about Emma and about the almost-upon-me transplant, in between trips to the bathroom to vomit. I was feeling for the first time the 'looseness' of being drunk. The alcohol numbed the pain in my heart, and yet brought me closer to it — drink made me talk about my emotions freely.

It was a good night. It was a heartbreaking night, too.

Two days after my first drinking binge, I had a new Broviac inserted. This catheter was identical to the old one. The new one, though, emerged from slightly higher above my right nipple. Just below the entry site of my new Broviac was the circular scar left by my old catheter.

After I had my Broviac inserted, I awoke to the knowledge that my six-and-a-half-year run as a Crumlin outpatient was at an end. The next time I entered the hospital, I didn't know how long I'd be staying for.

20 June 2001. A few days after my Broviac was put in, the date I'd been anticipating for months and months arrived.

My first port of call that morning was St Luke's Hospital in Rathgar, Dublin. It was there that I had my radiotherapy, or TBI — total body irradiation. The purpose of this radiotherapy was to destroy my own Fanconi-affected bone marrow, before the donor's healthy marrow was transplanted into me. The TBI would make it far more likely that the donor's marrow would 'engraft', or be accepted by my system.

It was strange to have this first act of my bone marrow transplant performed in a hospital other than Crumlin. Luke's was not a hospital exclusively for children, and so I found the atmosphere quite different from that of Our Lady's. As I walked through the corridors, flanked by my parents, I even thought it strange that the walls were decorated with works of modern art, rather than with murals of Disney characters.

Amidst all this colour, it was almost difficult to believe that I was about to begin the biggest fight of my life.

Mai, Des, and I made our way to the St Luke's radiotherapy department, and found seats in the waiting area. Presently, a nurse called my name, and I was led away from my parents. I was taken to a room where I was weighed and measured. It was explained to me that the smaller a body is, the more radiation it absorbs relative to bodyweight. My being weighed and measured would help the doctors determine the amount of radiation that should be fired at me in order for me to receive the standard 'absorbed dose'. The regime of radiotherapy/chemotherapy that I was heading into was, technically speaking, lethal. If I wasn't 'saved' by someone else's marrow, these 'therapies' would kill me.

After the weighing and measuring, I was led to a dressing room. I was asked to strip down to my underwear, and was given a blue 'theatre gown' to put on. Thanks to my many bone marrow aspirations, I was used to wearing these gowns. They were made from a material that felt like crepe paper, and they had to be tied at the back with papery strips.

Once I'd donned my gown, the nurse took me to a spacious grey room. There was a radiation screen dividing one part of this room from the rest, and there was a large machine in front of the screen. Directly opposite the machine was a rectangular glass box, lying on a platform. There were several medical personnel present in the room. Compared to these neatly dressed staff, I felt naked. The crepe-like gown didn't keep out the cold.

I was ordered to climb into the glass box. This I did. Then I lay still, listening to the tinkles of banal pop music that were coming from speakers in the ceiling. The medical staff went behind the protective screen, and the lights dimmed. Occasionally, a voice would ask me to turn one way or another, as the machine opposite me fired radiation at different sides of my body. Twenty or so minutes later, the TBI was over.

I went to my dressing room, pulled off my blue gown, and put back on the sweatshirt and tracksuit bottoms that I'd had for years. I returned to Mai and Des, and then a doctor took the three of us into a small office. This doctor began to describe the short-, medium-, and long-term side effects of radiotherapy.

I was told that, within a few hours, I would probably feel queasy and feverish. I would most likely develop high temperatures and severe diarrhoea within days. In about a fortnight, my hair would start to fall out. The dose of radiation I'd received increased my risk of getting assorted forms of cancer, and could lead to the growth of cataracts on my eyes. The operation to remove these cataracts might result in my having to choose either long-sightedness or short-sightedness for myself. The TBI, of course, also made me sterile.

A sort of numbness came over me as I left St Luke's Hospital on the morning of 20 June 2001. There was too much to feel, and all my emotions were trying to shove themselves into my soul, but none of them was making it because they were all battling against one another so hard. And so I just felt numb. Steeled. Ready for unknown trials.

This was it.

Mum, Dad, and I pulled into the car park at Our Lady's Hospital for Sick Children at around lunchtime. The three of us approached the main hospital entrance, preparing to plod the familiar walk to St John's Ward.

I paused just before entering the hospital, and let my parents move a few steps ahead. I looked out over the car park, and breathed in deeply. I knew this would be my last breath of fresh air for a long time.

'Ben?' my mum called, from beyond the hospital doors.

I turned. 'I'm coming,' I said.

12. Hell, part one

The High Dependency Unit of St John's Ward was exactly the way I remembered it. The unit had three 'ordinary' isolation rooms and two 'transplant' rooms. There was also a toilet/shower room. Two sets of red double doors led into the unit, which still had — like the rest of St John's — that blue linoleum floor and those beige walls. At the top of the HDU was the conservatory in which Dr Breatnach told my parents that I had FA. A door led from the conservatory out to the Crumlin Hospital staff car park.

My parents and I entered the HDU through the two sets of double doors, and were welcomed by a nurse. I immediately got a sense of how in-demand this place was. The nurse snapped a bracelet with my name and hospital number on it around my wrist, and then I had to sit and wait for more than an hour, until a room became free. Another transplant patient was just leaving.

When my room became available, I was taken to it. I'd be spending my first five days here, in one of the ordinary isolation rooms, having chemotherapy. The purpose of the chemo was to supplement the radiotherapy; it would ensure that my own bone marrow was utterly destroyed, and that my immune system was as suppressed as it could be, before I received the new marrow.

In a twist of fate which brought a smile to my face, the ordinary isolation room I was shown into was the same room that I'd been in when I spent those days in the HDU in November-December 1993.

There had been some debate, before my admission to St John's, about whether I should have my transplant in Crumlin or in St James's Hospital, a few miles away. The facilities in James's were more modern, and better suited to 'young adults'. But in the end I'd decided to have my BMT in Our Lady's, simply because I knew the doctors and nurses. The type of bone marrow transplant I was about to undergo was a new kind of transplant, and I was going to become the first person in Ireland to have it. This new kind of BMT involved a revolutionary immunosuppressant drug called fludarabine. One of the biggest fears during a BMT, and particularly during a BMT involving a donor who is not related to the patient, is that the patient will develop graft versus host disease, or GVHD. GVHD is when the donor's marrow attacks the patient's tissues and organs; in milder cases, the disease results in a rash akin to acute sunburn; in more serious cases, GVHD can lead to stomach, liver, and intestinal damage, and can even be fatal. In twenty-four trial matched unrelated donor transplants in the United States involving FA patients and fludarabine, the instances of GVHD had been significantly reduced.

Twelve of these patients died anyway, however, due to other transplant complications.

I thought about this statistic as I settled into the place that was going to be my home for an uncertain amount of time.

In order to take my mind off morbid thoughts, as my parents and I unpacked my bags, I pretended that I was moving into a hotel. After all, I was going to have my meals brought to me; my room had a television in it — and the hospital had more TV channels than we had at home; plus, I'd brought my stereo and my Dreamcast games machine. I also had a freshly purchased laptop, as well as books, magazines, CDs.

There were cupboards in my room, and my parents and I put all my stuff into these. The only other piece of furniture the room contained, apart from the bed, was a blue leather armchair. This chair rested by the large window that looked out onto the grassy hospital grounds.

As time went by, Mai or Des could be found sitting in this armchair for hours each day, while I lay or sat up in my bed. One of my parents was by my side constantly. Every night, either Mum or Dad stayed in one of the parents' rooms in Our Lady's. Sometimes, during the day, both Mai and Des were with me. When this was the case, a relative or friend took care of Ruth and Jess. Des spent so much time in Crumlin during the summer of 2001 that he joined a gym around the corner from the hospital. Mai's friends would occasionally meet her for breakfast or lunch in the hospital canteen. My parents often drove to Crumlin by different routes; they'd compare notes and between them try to find the quickest route from Kilmacanogue to Our Lady's.

On that first day, I nestled as well as could be expected into my isolated surroundings. The sweet illusion of living in a hotel, however, dissolved pretty rapidly. Soon after my arrival at the HDU, a nurse came to hook me up, via my Broviac, to the chemo, and to other IV medications.

As well as intravenous meds, I was given many pills. As the days went by, the number of tablets I had to take continued to increase, until I was on over thirty a day — all different kinds, all different shapes and sizes; some of the pills looked like sweets, others like bits of chalk. Tablets were delivered to me in a silver cup each morning, lunchtime, teatime, and bedtime.

My first night in the HDU in June 2001 went by without drama. Things were going swimmingly until the predictions of the TBI doctor came true. On the day after I was admitted to Crumlin, I started to suffer rigors and spiking temperatures. And man, did I experience diarrhoea. Litres of black liquid began flowing out of me — it was like I was an oil well. Overnight, I also became cripplingly weak. Too weak to even walk across the corridor to the toilet. Every half-hour or so, a commode had to be wheeled into my room for me. When I just needed to pee, a nurse or one of my parents would bring me a transparent plastic pee bottle.

During the next few days, I spent most of my time in bed, dressed only in boxer shorts and a t-shirt. Usually, I was asleep; when I was awake, I was barely so. I was zonked from the radiotherapy, the chemo, the drugs.

Each morning, I was just about able to potter across to the shower, to let the warm water ease my tensions. Hygiene is even more important during transplant than it is normally.

On occasion during that first week of my BMT, neighbours or friends of the family would arrive at Our Lady's to see my parents. These neighbours or friends would then walk around the side of the hospital, and look in at me through my room's large window. This was all they could do. To protect me from infection, no one was supposed to have access to my room except the medical staff, my parents, and another designated person — in my case, my aunt Bing. I was touched by the kindness of these visitors to my window; it was impossible not to be — even if their gawking did make me feel a little like a zoo exhibit.

While the 'no undesignated persons' rule was generally strictly obeyed, sometimes exceptions were made. One day during that first week, for example, Dr O'Marcaigh gave two of my good friends since BSP days special permission to come into my room to chat with me. I had thought I wouldn't be able to see any of my friends until the transplant was over, so it really was a terrific surprise when my two BSP pals walked through the door. One mate joked that he'd smuggle me in some booze if I smuggled him out some drugs. I laughed. My friends' presence perked me up a bit.

I needed perking up. By Saturday 23 June, my weakness had become totally overpowering. I had headaches, stomachaches, a raised heart rate and high blood pressure. I also couldn't sleep. I couldn't do anything else, either — because I was too sick and weak. I just had to lie there, my body drained and painful, my mind racing.

On Sunday 24 June, my morning blood test revealed that my counts were extremely low. That afternoon, I was given a transfusion.

Then, on the evening of 24 June, I had my first nasogastric (NG) tube inserted.

'Which nostril do you want it in?' a nurse asked.

I volunteered my left.

The end point of the tube was pushed up my nose. I was told to keep swallowing through the ticklish, painful sensation, as the tube was slipped down my throat. I gagged, but I continued to swallow — and soon, one end of the NG tube was in my tummy. To make sure of this, the nurse attached a syringe to the other end, and sucked some juices up from my stomach. The end of the tube that wasn't in my tummy was then taped to the side of my face.

The nasal tube could be used to send liquid medicines directly to my stomach, without my having to endure their foul tastes. Two days later, however, in a fit of vomiting, I puked up my NG tube, and had to go through the process of having one slipped into my tummy all over again. It was the first of several times that happened.

On my fifth day in Crumlin, I had to have a CT scan done of my brain. This was in order to make sure I had no neurological problems. The scan, thankfully, came back clear.

The next day, Dr Gina MacDonnell visited me. I didn't say much to Gina. But, when she left me, the psychologist told my parents I seemed to be of sound mind.

That, at least, is always good to hear.

Later that evening, I was moved out of my ordinary isolation room, and taken across to one of the transplant rooms. The new location was about half the size of the previous one. I still had a television, though. Plus, the transplant room came equipped with its own phone line.

The benefits of being in the transplant room ended there, however. Concerns about hygiene and pathogens were even higher when a patient was in this room. For that reason, only items which could be wiped down with alcohol were allowed in the transplant room. This meant I couldn't have books or magazines. My clothes, of course, couldn't be wiped with alcohol, but they had to be washed at sixty degrees Celsius after each wear.

The transplant rooms were also known as 'laminar flow rooms'. This name came from the laminar airflow units that were used to purify the air in these rooms, and to keep out airborne infections. Neither transplant room had a door—each was separated from the rest of the HDU by a curtain and a yellow line. Before a nurse or parent crossed over this line, he or she had to don a plastic apron. All surfaces in the laminar flow rooms also had to be scrubbed with alcohol wipes daily, to ensure no dust settled and no germs grew.

At 8.30 p.m. on Tuesday 26 June 2001, Dr Aengus O'Marcaigh arrived at my bedside. He was about to perform possibly the most important act of my life.

My new marrow had been harvested from my American donor less than twenty-four hours earlier. The marrow had then been collected from a hospital in the US by one of the St John's nurses, who'd taken a flight straight back to Ireland with it.

As I lay in bed that Tuesday evening, I thought of my anonymous donor. He or she was willing to undergo a painful bone marrow harvest, in order to save the life of an Irish teenager he or she didn't know. It was astonishing to think that I was about to become so profoundly connected to someone I had never even met. I wondered about my donor's interests, his or her hobbies, what he or she liked to eat for breakfast.

A bone marrow transplant is not like a heart transplant or a lung transplant. For one thing, obviously, the donor doesn't have to die before he or she can save the life of another. And, for the recipient, there is no surgical operation. A friend once told me that he thought I had all my bones sliced open, my old marrow scooped out, and my new marrow stuffed in. Nothing as dramatic as that took place.

The actual transplant itself was about as undramatic as it gets.

I sat on the edge of my bed, and Aengus attached a six-inch-long syringe filled with clear liquid to one of the three small tubes at the end of my Broviac. This clear liquid was a suspension of blood-cell-creating stem cells. These stem cells had been purified from the donor's harvested marrow — they were, in effect, my new marrow, purified. Ever so slowly, Aengus pushed my new stem cells into me.

The procedure was painless, and lasted just ten minutes.

When all of the suspension was inside me, coursing through my veins and finding its way to my bones, Mai, Des, and I shook hands with Aengus.

He smiled, but warned that the toughest times were ahead.

And so the waiting began.

Throughout the days immediately after receiving the donor's stem cells, I felt a little better than I had done the previous week. I was still overwhelmed by tiredness, but I wasn't quite as sick. I entertained myself by browsing the Internet on my laptop (courtesy of the phone socket in the laminar flow room), or by playing my Dreamcast. I tried to keep up my regular television schedule as well, watching the programmes I'd normally have watched at home — *The West Wing*, *The Practice*, any programme, really, about American politics or American lawyers.

While I was in the transplant room, personal hygiene became more difficult. I had to wash daily, but I wasn't allowed to leave the protective environment of my room — even to go to the shower. So, every morning, my mum or my dad would bring me in a basin filled to the brim with lukewarm water. I'd stand in the basin and dab myself down with a facecloth. After I'd done this and re-dressed myself, I'd call Mai or Des back in to wash my hair. I'd kneel over the basin while Mum or Dad scrubbed my scalp. I felt like a baby again.

The days continued to drift by, and my health began to worsen once more. Eating became a chore, especially with the NG tube down my throat — I could feel it inside me every time I swallowed. Therefore, I was put on a liquid, high-energy, nutrient-rich feed, which was administered via my NG tube. A litre of the stuff took about two hours to go in.

One afternoon, I was sitting in the blue leather armchair in the laminar flow room. My nasal tube was connected up to an NG feed pump, and the machine was gradually pushing feed into me. The pump, however, was over the other side of the room (it wasn't a very big room), and the tubing connecting it to my nose was running above the floor at about ankle height. My mum was walking over to me, when she stepped on the tubing. The NG tube flew out of my stomach, up through my throat, and out my nose — spraying sticky beige feed everywhere, making me vomit all over the floor.

'Jesus!' Mai exclaimed.

Despite the fact that I had just puked, and that my NG tube had come up and I would have to suffer having another one put down, I erupted in laughter.

That wasn't the only humorous incident that took place during my BMT.

Just inside the entrance to the High Dependency Unit, there was a telephone with its own extension number. This phone was for parents; they could use it to make calls, and if they gave the extension number to friends or relations, mums and dads could receive calls on this phone, too.

One evening, the HDU phone rang, and Des went to pick it up.

'Hello?' my dad said.

'Hi,' a woman's voice with an English tint replied. 'I was just wondering, what kind of package holidays do you offer? I'm thinking I'd like to go to Majorca. Now —'

'I'm sorry,' Des interrupted, 'you must have the wrong number.'

How on earth does someone intending to contact a travel agency end up phoning the High Dependency Unit of a children's hospital?

When Dad came back to my room and told me this story, I couldn't stop laughing. I felt about as far from the sun and sand of a summer holiday as it was possible to feel.

One morning around a fortnight after my total body irradiation, I awoke in my bed in the laminar flow room. I lifted my head from my pillow, and discovered I'd left hair on its white surface. I pulled at the locks on my scalp, and found that they slid out easily.

Within days, all of my hair, all over my body, had been shed. I felt strangely prepubescent without it.

On 4 July, the results of one of my routine blood tests indicated that the engraftment of the donor marrow was going well. My blood counts were rising.

I was still having transfusions of blood and platelets regularly, however, in order to boost my counts, and in order to prevent excessive bleeding or bruising.

The number of medications I had to take kept increasing as well. I was on a host of antibiotics and other drugs, all designed keep away infection and GVHD.

When I felt able to eat, the food I was given did not come from the regular canteen, but was specially prepared under strict hygiene conditions. My parents weren't even permitted to bring me food from home.

As the early days of July ticked by, and as my counts rose, I did begin to feel a little less poorly. Some afternoons, I was even well enough to be bored, and wondered when I was going to be let out of my damn prison cell. Dr O'Marcaigh, however, continued to caution my incredulous parents and me that my sickest days were to come.

July turned into its second week, and I became unbelievably sleepy once again. I tried to keep up my routine of television, videogames, and emails but I often just nodded off.

At times I seemed to ramble and become incoherent. One afternoon, I said to my mother, 'I saw someone on TV walk once — I tried to copy them.'

On 10 July, I was shifted from the laminar flow room back to my ordinary isolation room. This meant that my counts were high enough for me to be afforded certain privileges again — such as having access to books, and being allowed to shower.

Despite these higher blood counts, however, I didn't feel stronger. I felt frailer than ever. The drugs were wiping me out, and I was beginning to suffer muscle wastage from all the time I was spending in bed.

On the morning of Friday the 13th, I pottered across to the shower room for my daily wash. I shut the door, and took off my t-shirt and boxer shorts. As I undressed, I couldn't help noticing my body in the mirror above the sink on the opposite wall.

My scalp was cracked and red; the rest of my skin was as dry as my forehead had been during First Year. My limbs were pale sticks; I'd lost a lot of weight, but my stomach and face appeared bloated. I thought I looked like the kind of man a child might draw: a big circle for a torso, a small circle for a head, and four straight thin lines for arms and legs.

I'd never really liked the way I looked before my transplant. But now I hoped I would one day look like that again.

I turned away from the mirror, and switched on the shower. This shower was part of the room itself; the water fell down onto the floor, and drained away through a hole.

I began to wash myself. I scrubbed my chest and my stomach with a sponge.

Suddenly, things became yellower than they should have been. And then I felt myself falling.

When my consciousness fogged back into place several seconds later, water was trickling across my face. I knew from the pain that I had bruised myself badly.

I moved my arm to try and hoist myself onto my knees. But I wasn't able to lift my own body weight. My face again hit the wet beige floor.

I pushed a button to alert the nurses that I needed help. Two came sprinting in. Between them, the nurses got me back on my feet. They dried me with a coarse white towel, helped me put on a clean t-shirt and clean boxers, and escorted me back to my room.

The humiliation of this incident left me feeling horribly ashamed and sorry for myself. I was a sixteen-year-old boy. I was supposed to be growing independent. Yet with each passing day, I was becoming more and more dependent on others.

There is an old hospital adage, which one of the nurses in St John's related to me once: When you go into hospital, you take two suit-cases with you — one to carry your clothes, and another to pack away your dignity. Certainly, there was no place for petty pride in the High Dependency Unit. After my fainting episode, I didn't want to have any more showers, in case I fell again. After I collapsed in the shower a second time a few days later, I usually settled for bed baths — I'd scrub myself down with a warm, wet facecloth, while lying in bed. As my energy waned, even the task of giving myself a bed bath became insuperable. Mai, Des, or a nurse had to do it for me. I still insisted on washing my own groin and bottom, though. I had to retain some privacy.

But retaining privacy became tougher as I grew ever weaker.

Though it had improved since the opening weeks of the BMT, my diarrhoea was still with me. Sometimes I'd wake up to find myself squirming in my own shit. One morning, I remember, a nurse came into my room with my first course of pills for the day. I had just woken up, and I knew I had soiled my boxers. Neither of my parents had arrived yet, and I couldn't climb out of bed. So I asked this nurse if she would be able to get me a clean pair of underwear. I pointed to the cupboard that my underwear was in, and she opened it. There were two bags in the cupboard; one of them was full of clean boxers, the other of dirty boxers. I didn't know which was which. The nurse dipped her hand into one of the bags, yanked out a pair of boxers, tossed it to me, and then left the room. I looked at the boxers. The inside of them was coated in shit. But they were at least in better shape than the pair I had on. So I slowly pulled off that pair and put on the 'new' pair.

Diarrhoea didn't just show up in my boxers in the morning. Around ten times a day, I needed to sit on the commode—while my arse basically exploded. My behind became so red and sore that I had to wipe it with soft gauze and olive oil rather than toilet paper. Cream was used to ease my anal agitation, as well. Once daily, a nurse would come into my room, don latex gloves, then stick her finger between my bum cheeks and rub the white cream around my arsehole.

When I had to use the commode, I would tell whichever parent was with me, and then Mai or Des would fetch the toilet-on-wheels. Mai or Des would then leave the room, pulling across all the curtains as they did so. When I'd done my business and was back in bed, I'd yell that I was finished. Mum or Dad would step into my room again, and whisk away the commode.

One evening while Des was with me, however, I called out to him before I was back under the covers. Des, who was standing just outside my room, opened the door to find me struggling to lift myself off the commode. Brown trickles of shit were running down my legs.

Des shouted for a nurse, and one came. She cleaned my legs and wiped my bum, then tucked me back in beneath the bed sheets.

I cried.

I'd become too weak to even wipe my own behind.

By 18 July, my condition had deteriorated greatly. I was flitting in and out of consciousness. My kidneys were poor. I had aches all over. My diarrhoea had worsened, and I was now sleeping atop an incontinence mat. Blood and sugar were appearing in my stools and urine, as well.

Dr O'Marcaigh told my parents that my system appeared to be breaking down.

When I was awake, I couldn't see very well. As days passed, my vision became increasingly blurred, till I could make out only the outline of shapes. I was wheeled through the hospital corridors, with a mask over my face, to visit an ophthalmologist. She, however, couldn't see any solution to my problem.

To make matters worse, my ears were stuffed with wax, and I was finding it hard to hear. Plus, my nose was clogged with so much hardened gunge that I couldn't breath through it. Breathing through my mouth wasn't easy either, as the insides of my cheeks were lined with stinging blisters.

What's more, my weight loss was becoming uncontrollable. I was now being fed via total parenteral nutrition, or TPN — i.e. intravenously.

Eventually, a doctor came and unblocked my nose; using a special pair of tweezers, he pulled shards of bloody red-green snot out of my nostrils. Then another doctor arrived to syringe my ears. So my breathing problem and my hearing problem, at least, were cleared up.

One afternoon around this time, Gina arrived for another chat with me. I told her that I was scared of losing my sight, that it was so frustrating to be attached to so many machines. She seemed to think that, despite it all, mentally, I was coping well.

The days ticked on, and I started to pee blood constantly. I was now incontinent, and there was no telling when a stream of red piss was going to come out of me and ruin my lovely white bed sheets. Once, Mai changed my bedclothes sixteen times in twelve hours.

Up to that point, I'd continued to insist on getting out of bed to pee into a pee bottle. But now I had no choice but to have a catheter inserted. The tube would go into my bladder through my urethra, and draw all my urine into a bag. The bag could rest on the side of my bed, or be carried with me if I had to go anywhere.

Early one July night, a middle-aged doctor I hadn't met before arrived to put in my catheter. My parents left the room, and the doctor sat by the edge of my bed. I tossed back the sheets, and slipped my boxers down to around my knees.

The doctor took my penis in his gloved hand. He pushed the tip of the catheter into the slit at the top of my organ.

The pain was startling.

It got worse as he forced the tube further down my urethra. I could feel the thing moving inside me. Tubes aren't supposed to go there.

The next morning, my sheets were still stained with pee. Would you believe—the catheter hadn't been put in properly. After three days, it fell out, and a new one had to be inserted.

That second catheter stayed in, thankfully. And it was actually handy, as it kept the bedclothes clean. But while it was inside me, I never lost the sensation of needing to pee. I couldn't tell when I was peeing and when I wasn't.

And the catheter caused such appalling pain—the worst physical pain I've ever felt in my life. Its presence exacerbated the infection-pains I was already feeling in my groin.

During Fourth and Fifth Class, I used to get cramps in my feet. These cramps had often reduced me to wriggling on the floor. But the pain from them was like brushing against feathers compared to what I was going through now.

Now, it was as though my whole groin had been set alight; or as if there were a little man inside my penis, repeatedly stabbing me.

I spent days just squirming in my hospital bed, trying to free myself from the agony.

But it didn't go away.

On 21 July 2001, after weeks of having erratic blood sugars, I was declared diabetic, and placed on intravenous insulin.

I now needed so many IV medicines, that the three tubes of my Broviac were constantly in use—and I had a cannula in each arm, as well.

In order to take my daily blood test, doctors had to resort to pricking my thumb and squeezing the blood out. I was given so many thumb pricks during this period, however, that the tips of both my thumbs became infected. At the top of each, a tumescent, painful blister grew. These blisters looked like miniature blood-red balloons. And it was weeks before a doctor came to burst the blisters and bandage my thumbs.

On 26 July, a test result came back, and this test result confirmed that a viral infection had caused many of my recent problems — the blood in my urine, and so on.

Slowly, with the aid of medication, the virus was destroyed, and the pain in my groin faded.

But then I developed a sinus infection, and began to have nosebleeds.

And then one of my Broviac lines became infected, and the doctors had to rely more on my cannulae.

I was still losing weight; I still had the tube in my nose, the diarrhoea, the diabetes, the blurred vision. And I was still too weak to walk.

As July was taking its final bow, I asked the medical staff if there was anything I could do to strengthen my atrophied muscles. I must be able to help myself somehow, I thought.

And there was something I could do. A young physiotherapist named David came to see me, and he showed me how to perform bed exercises that would build up my leg and arm strength. David also suggested that it would be good for me to get out of bed and sit in the blue leather armchair in my room, at least for half an hour or an hour every day. The physiotherapist advised me to potter up and down the corridor of the HD Unit as often as I could, as well — to get used to the rhythm of walking again.

Each day from then on, David called to my room, and I did exercises with him. And, every day, he would leave me sitting in the blue armchair, rather than lying in bed. Never before had I found sitting so tiring; just being semi-upright seemed to make all my energy fall out of me. And I could almost hear my body creak as I lowered myself into and got up from the chair.

My body also seemed to creak as I ambled up and down the HDU corridor. I would take awkward, off-balance steps, pushing my IV pump with one hand, and carrying the bag attached to my urinary catheter in the other.

Gradually but progressively, my health improved. My vision came back into focus; the diarrhoea eased off; the sores in my mouth shrivelled away; my blood sugars settled down and my IV insulin was halted; I stopped peeing blood and my catheter was taken out. My cannulae were also removed. My nasogastric tube was left in, but I returned to eating solid food. I stopped haemorrhaging weight. I started reading books again, watching TV, listening to the radio, to my CDs.

But I had lost all desire to leave hospital. I was frightened. I had become institutionalised, addicted to my routine. Each morning, I looked forward religiously to my breakfast of scrambled eggs on toast. After breakfast, I looked forward to dinner. Then I looked forward to my tea. What else was there to look forward to but mealtimes?

The 1st of August 2001 was a momentous day in the course of my bone marrow transplant. Dr Fin Breatnach, acting as captain of my BMT ship while Aengus was on holiday, allowed me to go home — if only for a few hours.

I was anxious about spending even one afternoon out of the hospital. But the medical staff seemed to think it would be healthy for me to start re-familiarising myself with my old environment.

So I donned a protective mask, and sat in a wheelchair. Mai pushed me up the HDU corridor and out the conservatory door. The nurses waved goodbye.

It was odd to be in the car again, making that all-too-familiar journey across the Dublin Mountains to Kilmac.

When we got to our house, I noticed one big change. My parents had decided to get rid of most of the patio on which Emma and I had performed 'Thriller' four years before. They were now building a sunroom on this site. Construction hadn't finished yet, and what would one day be a sunroom was for the moment just a wet, grey shell. It was hard to imagine the shell as a completed conservatory.

I wasn't allowed to go near the under-construction sunroom; the disturbed soil and all the filthy concrete no doubt contained millions and millions of deadly germs. I spent the afternoon in my own bed, reading the fourth Harry Potter book for the second time.

My room was not in the state I had left it six weeks previously. It'd had to be thoroughly cleaned before I arrived home, so, Mai and a friend of hers had taken everything off my shelves, dusted the shelves and wiped them down. All my boxes of CDs, videos, etc. were now piled up in the hall outside my door. The sight of them almost made me despair. I liked to keep my stuff organised and accessible!

My mum cooked pasta for me that evening. After dinner, we drove back to Our Lady's.

Over the next few days, I left the High Dependency Unit a few more times. I visited my paternal grandparents; I went home again. One afternoon, Mai and Des took me to Powerscourt Waterfall in Wicklow — the place of many a happy childhood walk. We couldn't get out of the car, however, as there was a thunderstorm crackling across the sky; sheets of rain were turning the landscape into a soaked sponge.

So I sat in the back seat and laughed. Somehow, in spite of the greyness of the day, it was refreshing to just sit and look at the white, gushing waterfall, the rusting autumn trees.

I was amidst natural beauty again. And it beat the sterility of the HDU any day.

On Thursday 9 August 2001, I was discharged from Crumlin Hospital. I was still taking over two dozen pills per day; I still had my nasogastric tube and my Broviac. Dr Breatnach, however, felt my condition would improve quicker at home.

My mum was handed a timetable detailing when all of my tablets had to be taken, and was shown how to operate my NG tube. She already knew how to clean my Broviac, but she was given a quick revision course in this as well.

I said farewell to the nurses, knowing that, whatever happened, I would be back in the coming days for a blood test.

I sat serenely in the wheelchair as Mum wheeled me out the conservatory door, and I wondered what sort of life I was heading into.

13. Hell, part two

I did not feel ready to go home. I was nervous about being away from the safety of the hospital. To make matters worse, I felt sicker than I had in some time. The all-over aches had returned; my knees were particularly sore, and my eyes were excruciatingly bloodshot. My blood counts were lower than they'd been for weeks, as well. I had thought going home would mean I was completely better. I was far from completely better.

On the way back to Kilmacanogue, I listened to the car radio. A news presenter was chattering away. I'd always been interested in current affairs; from the age of ten, I was more likely to be found watching the news than watching cartoons. Now, however, events in the wider world seemed utterly detached from me, from my cocoon of a life. I almost thought I should be hearing about my personal progress on the bulletins.

When Mai and I arrived at our house, I went to my room. I just lay on my bed, and hoped that my tears would fall. But I was so deadened, I couldn't even cry.

On Saturday 11 August, I puked up my nasogastric tube. A rush of relief drowned my anxiety. Now they'll have to take me back, I thought.

My mum drove me to the HDU on Saturday afternoon. But the Crumlin team refused to readmit me. I sat in the conservatory while a nurse put a new nasogastric tube down my throat, and a doctor drew a blood sample from my Broviac. Then Mai and I went home.

That night, I didn't sleep at all. Mum sat by my bed till dawn broke.

On Sunday morning, I vomited up my tube again. Mai called the hospital, and one of the nurses told her to leave the tube out, and see how I fared solely on solid food.

I then discovered why it was a good idea to use the nasal tube to administer liquid oral medications. Without the NG tube, I was forced to squirt syringe-fuls of vile-tasting medicine into my mouth several times daily. My tongue burned for minutes after each dose.

On Monday 13 August, Dr O'Marcaigh — fresh back from his holidays — phoned. He told Mai that Saturday's blood test had revealed the presence of CMV in my system. I was to be readmitted to Crumlin immediately.

CMV, or cytomegalovirus, is a common infection among BMT patients. It affects some thirty per cent of people undergoing a BMT, and usually develops during the second or third month following the actual transplant. It can be fatal.

As soon as I got back to St John's, I was hooked up to an intravenous drip containing ganciclovir, a drug used to combat CMV.

I sat in the HDU conservatory for most of that afternoon. As the day went on, Mai noticed that I was becoming increasingly agitated and confused. She was alarmed at how quickly this was happening, and spoke to Aengus about it. Aengus, however, claimed he wasn't worried.

My confusion, though, kept worsening. Within twenty-four hours, I seemed to have lost all association with reality.

Gina came to see me on Wednesday 15 August. She sat beside the bed in my room. I lay in the bed, my eyes dull as stones.

'How are you?' the psychologist asked.

'I like trees,' I replied.

'Why do you like trees, Ben?'

'They do good things,' I said, 'unlike people.'

Gina nodded, as if this were a perfectly normal conversation we were having.

Over the next few days, my mind constructed a nightmare life for me. My parents were dead. They'd been killed in a car accident. The rest of my family had died in a plane crash. I'd been sent to a juvenile home, and tied to my bed. Because of all the tubes coming out of me, it wasn't difficult to imagine that I was strapped down.

My brain even interpreted normal situations in terrifyingly bizarre ways. One afternoon, Aengus came to visit me. I saw him deathly grey, with water falling from him onto the floor. This was because my mind told me he'd drowned himself the previous night. I freaked—it was his ghost!

I heard constant screaming. I saw the baby in the room beside mine being beaten and stabbed by nurses.

One night, masked men burst into my room.

Another night, I yanked at the tubes coming from my chest, then rang the bell for a nurse.

When the nurse came, I said, 'I have to relieve the pressure.'

'What do you mean, Ben?' she asked.

I didn't know what I meant.

'It's just . . .' I went on, struggling under the covers, 'the pressure . . . I have to get rid of it.'

Throughout this psychotic episode, I was hardly eating anything. The food that I did consume, I puked up within hours. One morning, a nurse tried to put an NG tube down my throat.

I was having none of it.

'Fuck off!' I shrieked. 'Get that fuckin' thing away from me!'

I pushed and squirmed. I wouldn't stop. Scared and exasperated, the nurse gave up.

After visiting me on Wednesday the 15th, Gina had concluded that my psychosis was a neurological problem. She sent a neurologist to see me.

I thought this neurologist was a man from the FBI.

The man from the FBI asked me to remember three words — 'world', 'watch', and 'blue'.

I remembered these words. I clung to them. My life depended on 'world', 'watch', and 'blue' — that much I was sure of.

But these three words, and my name, were all I could remember.

One evening, I opened my eyes from a stupor to see my mum leaning over me, tears trickling down her cheeks.

'Who're you?' I asked.

Another evening, my dad placed his hand on my shoulder as he left my room.

I recoiled. 'Don't touch me!' I said.

'Why not?'

'Every bone in my body is broken.'

Hospital procedure in Our Lady's can be frustrating. Sometimes waiting seems to be the only thing that gets done.

But things happen quickly in an emergency. And my parents later revealed to me that, during those psychotic days, they thought I was going to die. My mum once walked into my room, and I was so unresponsive she thought I was dead.

After the neurologist saw me, I was rushed up to theatre to have a lumbar puncture. This was to check my spinal fluid and make sure there was nothing wrong with my central nervous system. Thankfully, my CNS was okay.

Two days later, I was put in an ambulance, and it sped off across Dublin City. I was going to Beaumont Hospital—I needed an emergency MRI scan, and Our Lady's didn't have an MRI machine. Mai, Des, and a nurse came with me in the ambulance. The only thing I remember is a voice wondering if we were travelling too fast. It was my mum's. The driver assured her that he was going at a safe speed, as he weaved in and out of speeding traffic.

The purpose of the MRI was to determine whether the cytomegalovirus had reached my brain. If it had, there was little hope of my recovery.

But it had not.

When I returned, heavily sedated, to Our Lady's, a psychiatrist named Neil Adamson came to see me. Dr Adamson and Gina agreed that my psychosis had been caused by the ganciclovir. Psychosis was a recognised side effect of the drug, and mine had come on quickly and strongly after my first dose. Dr Adamson prescribed me an antipsychotic—Melleril. I took my Melleril pill daily.

Over the next few days, I developed a shake that would stay with me for weeks, and I wandered in and out of consciousness.

One day, my eyes opened just a little, and I thought I saw the blurred figures of my godfather, Kevin Hayes, and his wife, Anne, sitting in my room. Kevin looked across at me, and noticed that my eyes were open. Tiredness overpowered me, and the blurred figures disappeared into blackness.

By 29 August, the Melleril seemed to be taking effect. I continued to ramble, but my parents were seeing glimpses of my old self. I recognised who they were, at least.

As August turned into September, my world started to resemble the real world again.

But the terror still wouldn't leave.

By 1 September, I was under pressure to get out of Crumlin. The medical team once again thought that I would make more progress at home. Plus, there were other patients waiting for my room.

I didn't want to go home—especially after my false start the month before. Aengus came to me, and he assured me that my bed was mine for as long as I felt I needed it.

One evening around this time, Dr Fin Breatnach paid me a visit. He just wanted to say hello — he had no medical reason for coming to see me. He sat on the side of my bed, and told me that I'd soon be out of Our Lady's and taking the world by storm.

I didn't want to take the world by storm. I wanted to rot into nothing. The idea of doing anything but hiding frightened me so much.

Come the second week of September, despite Aengus's assurances, the pressure really was on to get me out of hospital. So, one Tuesday afternoon, my parents collected up my things, and I prepared to abandon Crumlin again. Maybe this time, I'd only be back as an outpatient.

Mai packed away my meds, Des crammed my clothes into bags. Then, my parents went off to lunch. They left me sitting up in my hospital bed, with the radio that was atop my bedside cupboard switched on. I was half-listening to *Liveline* with Joe Duffy, on RTÉ Radio One. It was the usual stuff — people complaining about random issues. But then, Mr Duffy announced that some news had just come in from New York. *Liveline* went to an ad break. When the programme resumed, listeners were told that an aeroplane had hit one of the Twin Towers.

I turned off the radio. I hobbled over to the television, and switched it on. I saw those pictures we all saw — the proud North Tower of the World Trade Center, dark smoke billowing from its upper storeys into the sky. The news anchor didn't know if this was an act of terrorism or a freak accident. Then a plane flew into the South Tower, and reports came in of a jet crashing into the Pentagon in Washington, DC. All doubts vanished. I watched as tiny bodies fell from the crumbling towers. It was impossible to believe that I was seeing the end of so many of lives.

Mai arrived back from lunch, and as she opened my door, I said, 'The World Trade Center is collapsing.'

She thought I was having another hallucination. But I pointed to the TV.

Nurses bustled in and out of my room throughout the rest of the afternoon — giving me tablets, saying farewell. Some were scared and shaken by the day's events. Others seemed nonchalant. 'I suppose there'll be another war now,' said one.

As for me—I felt guilty. It was almost as if the turmoil and horror I'd felt over the previous month had suddenly been loosed upon an unsuspecting America. I was petrified. I didn't know what would become of the world, or of me.

It was 11 September, 2001. And I was going home.

14. Home

'You'll never go to school again,' I said to my sisters as we sat watching television, the day after my release from transplant. Of course they would. But the world didn't seem the place for it anymore.

The house I returned to was pretty much the same as the one I'd left a month before. My things had been put back on my shelves, though not in the places they had occupied pre-transplant. There were two other changes to the room I remembered, as well. My parents had brought in an old television, and they had wired up a phone socket beside my bed.

The sunroom whose construction had begun during the summer was still under construction. So I couldn't wander down that end of the building. Not that I felt like walking even that far. I just wanted to stay in bed. My whole body complained painfully if I did anything else. Every part of me felt utterly shattered.

On the afternoon of my return to Kilmacanogue, Mai came into my room with a scissors, and cut off the hospital band which had been around my wrist for three months.

'You're home now,' she said.

I was in my house, but it didn't feel like I was home.

The day after I arrived back in Kilmac, a friend rang me. He would later describe my voice on that phone call as being like that of a ghost.

'So, you made it through?' my friend half-asked, half-stated.

I thought I would cry as I answered, 'Yeah.' It didn't seem like I'd made it through. It felt as though each week of the transplant had stripped away something of my insides, and now I was just a smashed, useless shell of a person.

One evening not too long after my friend's phone call, my mum asked me how I was doing.

I struggled for words. 'If there was an easy way to kill myself,' I said, 'I'd kill myself.'

Mai put her arms around me, and we stayed like that until our tears flowed.

Nights were the worst times. I often got no sleep at all. When I did, I just drifted in and out of horrific dreams for two or three hours. I imagined an immense darkness chasing me, hunting me down wherever I went.

The days were not much better. I was constantly attacked by irrational worries about the future — thoughts kept buzzing in and out of my head so rapidly, it was impossible to focus on any one thing. Did my friends still care about me? How was I going to catch up on my schoolwork? How was I going to learn to drive? Who was I going to marry?

I suffered terrible short-term memory loss, as well. I would put something somewhere, and then forget what I had done with it.

And beneath all this, I knew I was never going to get better.

Perhaps what scared me the most was the fact that I had lost my sense of things. I'd lost senses I thought I would never lose.

My sense of humour had disappeared. I didn't know why things were supposed to be funny. I was watching a movie in bed one afternoon and, during one scene, I thought to myself, You would have found this funny before your transplant. You'd better laugh. So I laughed. And I laughed. I couldn't halt my humourless laughing. Then: You'd better stop, I chastised myself. Stop, you idiot, it's not meant to be that hilarious.

I'd lost my sense of music, too. Songs I knew I'd liked before my BMT, I didn't know why I liked them. I couldn't feel any of the emotions in them. Even Michael Jackson left me cold.

I couldn't sing, either. I could hardly string a coherent spoken sentence together, let alone remember a melody. Before my transplant, when I was at home alone, I used to sing a lot. I'd sing songs by MJ, Tracy Chapman, Buddy Holly, Bruce Springsteen — all my favourites. Even though I was just singing for myself, I practised the songs, and I performed them — as if to an audience. Without a script to learn, it was the closest I got to the thrill of the stage.

Of course, words have a music all of their own. And, by September 2001, writing was another skill that had abandoned me. Weakness, combined with my continuous shaking, ensured that I couldn't even hold a pen, never mind hold a thought long enough to scribble it on paper.

After I left Our Lady's, I was still on a lot of medication. Every day, I was given some two dozen pills, including Melleril. I was also given the intravenous ganciclovir, for the persistent cytomegalovirus. I was free of my nasal tube, of course, and I was able to consume food in the normal way. But there were certain types of food that I wasn't allowed to eat: yoghurts, fresh fruit, organic or free-range produce — anything that might contain a lot of bacteria. Takeaways were out. Loaves of bread had to be disposed of after a day. I could only eat stuff that had come in sealed packages. Fresh French bread and many other things that I enjoyed were off the menu. I didn't really care that I couldn't eat these things, however. I never felt like eating.

Even though I wasn't eating much, my stomach and face still looked bloated. I wouldn't allow anyone to take photographs of me in my puffy, dry-skinned, still-hairless state. I guess my streak of vanity was something I had not lost.

Hygiene continued to be exceptionally important during those first weeks back home. I was supposed to wash myself every morning. Some mornings, though, the effort of standing up in the shower, even for a few minutes, was too much. I would simply wet the towels, and pretend that I was clean.

Before I departed Crumlin, David the physiotherapist told me that it was vital I keep up my regime of bed exercise at home. As the days passed, however, it became easier to increase my strength by simply walking. I started out by hobbling around the corridors of our house. Then I was able to hobble up and down our driveway, then up and down the lane that led to our driveway.

Mai stayed at home with me during those days, while Des was at work and my sisters were at school. Mum looked after me. She prepared my meals, cleaned my Broviac, gave me my medications. The hospital team had given us a pump for administering the ganciclovir, and Mai had learned how to operate this pump.

Mai also helped me on my strolls. Every day, the two of us would amble up and down the tree-lined, tarmacadamed laneway leading to our house. Mai would hold my arm, take my baby steps with me.

Even as these strolls made me stronger, however, every step hurt.

My friends were learning to drive. I was learning to walk again.

If there's one thing I've discovered in my life, it's that what I know changes. Or rather, what I think I know changes. I will be sure that what I believe is fact, and then my surety will ebb away.

When I emerged from Our Lady's, I was certain that my life had nowhere to go but death.

I don't really know how I got better, or at what point the certainty of death slipped away, like a falling veil, to reveal a sky filled with stars of hope.

But I did get better; that veil did fall away.

Maybe the heart carries the body and the mind through their challenges.

I'm sure all the medications I was taking had some impact as well!

My daily walks, and David's bed exercises, improved my muscle power — I was soon able to move normally. As the weeks went by, my terror lessened, and I stopped taking Melleril. I was weaned off ganciclovir too, as all traces of CMV cleared from my system. The doses of my other medications were also reduced. The shaking stopped. The dryness of my skin eased. My hair started to grow back, and it was furiously curly, just as it had been in my early childhood — though this time my curls were brown, not white. It didn't take long for the curls to grow out, but they were fun while they lasted.

Today, it seems as if I just woke up one morning, and suddenly all the pieces of my life were back in place. But I assume getting better took longer than that.

I remember one afternoon, sitting in the HDU conservatory during one of my regular post-BMT blood-test sessions. The radio was on, and Michael Jackson's new single was playing. I realised that I could feel music again. A few weeks later, MJ released his first album since 1997. When my dad arrived home with my copy, I held it in my hands — I was so excited! The cover was white with a glinting silver edge. The name of the album? *Invincible.*

As October turned into November, I found that I was able to hold a pen again. In early November '01, I started creating two new editions of *Totally Fushed*. My dad photocopied these issues and posted the copies to everyone on the *TF* mailing list. The new issues weren't as good as some of the previous ones. The covers were now black and white rather than colour, and each mag was only twenty pages long, as opposed to the typical thirty. 'Okay, so we're a little slimmer and we've lost our colour,' I wrote in the editorial for the first new edition, 'but that's the way I came out of hospital.'

As autumn '01 became winter '01, I was still largely confined to the house, while my immune system continued to recover. All of my trips out were to Crumlin Hospital, and on these I had to wear a mask over my nose and mouth. Because I couldn't go and meet them, my friends had to come up and visit me. No more than a pair of pals were allowed visit at once. My pals told me about the woes of Fifth Year, and brought me cards and presents.

The kindness of people, in fact — people I knew well and people I didn't, during my transplant and during the aftermath — was incredible. While I was in hospital, my sisters sent me postcards every single day. Friends phoned the laminar flow room while I was there, sent me books and letters. The employees in my dad's office sent me a huge card. My St Andrew's form sent me a card. My form teacher called around to my house after I was released. My Fifth Class teacher lent me a selection of his CDs. My chiropodist arrived at our house one evening with fruit and sweets for me (I couldn't eat the fruit, but you know what they say about the thought being the thing that counts).

Those are just a few examples of people's kindness. There are so many more.

My first non-hospital-related trip out of the house after I was released from the HDU, was a trip to the movies. One afternoon in November 2001, Mai and I went to see *Harry Potter and the Philosopher's Stone*. By now, I was able to venture outside without donning a mask. I couldn't remain away from home for too long, though. And it was still critical that I not be around crowds. That afternoon, I waited in the car while Mai went into the cinema to ask if many were expected to turn up for the matinee. Mum returned several minutes later, and told me that it was safe to go inside. The only other people present at the showing of the first Harry Potter film that day were six or seven school kids. Obviously, Harry Potter was far more important than school!

I couldn't order popcorn or a soft drink, but it was still brilliant to watch a movie on the big screen for the first time since my BMT. In the darkness of the cinema, watching the giant screen, I felt as though I were in another world. And just the fact that I could be taken to that other world meant I was making progress in the real one.

Going on my first fun trip out of the house wasn't the only post-BMT milestone I reached in November '01. That month also marked my return to education. I still couldn't go back to school. But teachers began coming to my house to give me one-on-one lessons. St Andrew's arranged for me to get home-tutored in a number of subjects. I also got help with Maths from one of our neighbours, who was a lecturer in UCD. And a man named John Douglas, who was a retired teacher and a friend of the family, helped me with English.

The St Andrew's College timetable allowed Leaving Certificate students to study eight exam subjects. But I only took seven — and that was quite enough.

Before I began my Leaving Cert studies in November '01, several doctors advised me not to. They told me that I should spend a year recovering, and then enter Fifth Year in August 2002. But I would not be left behind by my friends. When August 2002 came around, I was going to enter Sixth Year with them.

Besides, doing schoolwork made me feel that I was getting better. There was a soothing normality to it. My teachers gave me essays and exam questions to do; these were assignments I had to complete every week. I couldn't sit around wallowing in my problems and writing self-pitying reflections all day long.

Throughout the winter of '01, my health improved unrelentingly. And on the day before New Year's Eve, I was put under general anaesthesia in Crumlin Hospital, in order to have my Broviac catheter removed. This procedure left another tiny pink crater of a scar on my chest — I now had matching chest scars, one for each of the two most difficult periods of my life.

After the procedure, I awoke in the recovery room. Beeps and whirrs were filling my ears. For a few seconds, I didn't know where I was, or what was happening.

Then I remembered.

'Oh, you're awake,' a nurse's voice came through the fog of wooziness. 'Are you okay there?'

'Yeah,' I managed, through the mask that was pumping oxygen into my nose.

A new year was about to begin. And I was okay.

'And how long have you had this illness, this cancer?' Pierce Brosnan asked me. I didn't tell him FA wasn't a cancer. In a more metaphorical sense, he was probably right.

Besides—you don't correct James Bond, especially when you're sitting in his personal dressing room. That's right—my transplant was over, my health was leaping forward, and now I was sitting opposite 007 himself! Brosnan was filming the movie *Evelyn* at Ardmore Studios in Bray, and a meeting had been arranged for me through a friend of a friend of my mum's.

I was a pretty big James Bond fan, so naturally meeting Pierce was fantastic! Brosnan told me that he was a James Bond fan too: 'It certainly pays the bills.' Pierce was suave and charming. He offered me coffee and spoke about his own family. He gave me a look at the script for the next 007 movie, then codenamed 'Bond XX'. He told me he'd have to shoot me once I was finished with it.

Mai came with me to meet Pierce, and she did most of the talking. She smiled manically and spouted high-pitched platitudes about life and Celebrity. I just sat there thinking, Yep, I'm in a room with 007.

My friends were all tremendously impressed that I had met Pierce. At first they didn't believe me, but then I wrote an article about my encounter for *TF*, and I included two photos of me and Pierce with my article. One of the pictures showed Pierce shaking my hand, and the other showed him with his arm around me. The difference between these positions convinced my friends that I hadn't just met a waxwork figure of Mr Brosnan!

By now, I was able to deliver copies of *TF* in person—at least to my Andrew's pals. In early 2002, I paid my first visit to St Andrew's College since the end of Fourth Year. I wasn't permitted to stay long. I didn't attend any classes; I just met with some teachers, and then chatted to my friends during lunch break.

It was strange to be back in Andrew's under these circumstances. I was technically still a student at the school, but I felt as if I were a visiting dignitary—or at the very least an esteemed past pupil. All the other students were wearing their school uniforms; I didn't have mine on. I was apart again, and yet I was the centre of attention. It was like being onstage.

During lunchtime with my friends, I realised that a lot had changed. Some of my friends were no longer friends with each other. Some of my friends had got girlfriends. I could only watch these changes like theatre, before going home to the safety of isolation. Even as I was able to go out into the world more and more, I wanted still more.

Having re-familiarised myself with the St Andrew's scene, when February 2002 arrived, I was looking forward to going to the fourteenth One-Act Drama Festival at the school. Some of my friends were involved in the Andrew's play, a production of William Seebring's comedy, *The Original Last Wish Baby*. This year's play was not being directed by Mr Friel, but by a new drama instructor — Kristian Marken.

Just a few days before the festival opened, however, I started to feel a bizarre and constant tingling under my skin on the right side of my stomach. Within forty-eight hours, this prickling had developed into vicious red blisters that spread halfway down my right leg, all across my groin, and halfway up my torso. My mum took me to Crumlin. I was diagnosed with shingles, and admitted to St John's.

When I was five, I'd had chickenpox. I'd had spots everywhere — even on the inside of my throat. The antibodies created after a dose of chickenpox would normally prevent a person from coming down with shingles. Now that I had new bone marrow, however, all my old antibodies were gone. Over the next two years, I would need to be given the MMR, and a couple of other standard vaccinations, again. In February 2002, however, my immune system was still too weak for me to receive them.

That month, shingles caused me to spend a week in hospital. The infection cleared up completely with treatment. But I missed the One-Act.

And if you've never had it, just so you know — shingles is astonishingly painful. It was like there was a many-toothed monster clinging by its teeth to my thigh, groin, and stomach. Whenever I moved, it felt as though the teeth were tearing at my flesh.

I wasn't in the High Dependency Unit during those February days. I had a room to myself in the regular part of the ward. My parents obviously spent a lot of time by my bedside, but it wasn't necessary for them to be as attentive to me as they'd been throughout my BMT. Spring rolled on and, after my brief bout of shingles, my health continued to jump from strength to strength.

Yet I was dogged by thoughts of things that had happened before my transplant. In particular, I was worried about where I stood with Emma. Had my pre-BMT confession killed our friendship? I hadn't seen her since my return from hospital. After my release, she'd sent me a 'get well soon' letter in which she jokingly laid claim to the dedication in my first book. But that was the last time I'd heard from her.

In those days directly after my release from Our Lady's, when tangible thoughts had been so difficult to grasp, there was one thing that was always at the back of my mind: I knew there was a girl I loved. I couldn't feel music, I couldn't feel humour, and I couldn't feel my love for Emma, either. But I knew it was there. And once my mental and physical condition began to improve, my feelings for Emma came raging back, like a river finally rejoining the sea. They took up the place in my soul that they'd occupied previously, and they again took up their place at the forefront of my daily thoughts.

At the beginning of 2002, I knew there were some issues that I needed to settle with Emma. I was haunted by the fact that she had never even wanted to talk about my confession, or about the emotions I held for her. So, in March, I sent her a text message, asking if we could discuss the way I felt.

Emma wrote back that the whole thing was 'unpleasant', and that she still didn't want to talk about it.

I probably should have given up then. But, like Aurora drawn toward the spindle, I just couldn't stop. Later that month, I penned a letter, and posted it to Emma. My missive was essentially a more longwinded version of my text message.

A couple of days passed. Then, the postman delivered a letter from Emma.

'I don't really know what I can say,' the letter began. 'I'd like you, firstly, to put yourself in my position. Your friend tells you that he wants you to love him because he is dying. You want the truth, then fine — I was put on the spot and I felt you had absolutely no right to do that. I'm so sorry if I came across a tad annoyed. You seem to be implying that I was ignorant not giving you a last chance at love because you were dying. What the fuck was I supposed to do, Ben?

'I suppose I should try to come up with better ways to console my friends. No, in fact, I should just stop trying to sound nice, cos — you know me — I'll only end up pissing them all off.

'I can't believe you put me in such a position and now you're giving out about the way I handled it.'

When I finished reading Emma's letter, I put it back in its envelope, and set it on my desk. Then I slowly lay down on the floor of my room, flat on my stomach. The thoughts of all the things I would never have — they had become a vice on my mind, crushing. I felt the hardness of the floorboards on my fingertips, and through the folds of my clothing. I tensed my muscles and stretched out my limbs; I needed to know that I could still feel every inch of myself, because it seemed like despair was the only thing running through my veins. My soul was a battleground; it had been for years, as I'd fought against such aching, gripping, crippling obsession. And now, the object of my obsession was throwing back in my face the moment when I'd been most honest with her.

The way I saw it, I'd never tried to manipulate Emma's feelings — I'd simply told her mine. And I only told her because, at the lowest moment of my life, I couldn't keep the truth inside any longer — I wanted to be honest with her, I didn't want to die without letting her know. To be accused of emotional blackmail was impossibly painful.

I didn't stay on the floor for long. After a few minutes, I stood up, went to my desk, and wrote Emma a furious response.

I wanted to hate her. I needed to hate her.

Like so many other letters addressed to the girl of my dreams, however, this missive remained unsent. Writing it drained away of most of my anger. When I was finished, I was left only with sadness.

I put my letter aside, and simply sent Emma another text message. I told her that if she wanted to talk to me about her side of the story, I would listen.

She didn't write back.

A few days after I received Emma's heartbreaking letter, one of my mates called. He told me he was planning on having a small get-together at his house later in the week, as his parents were away. He asked if I'd like to come over for a few cans. I said I would. I also knew that this friend partook of a little marijuana from time to time. He hung up the phone, and I immediately rang him back.

'Will there be anything else at this party you're having?' I cautiously asked.

'Would you like there to be something else?' my pal inquired.

'I wouldn't mind,' I said.

'I'll see what I can do.'

On the night of the gathering, I got extremely drunk. Then I got stoned off my head for the first time in my life. When the weed was gone, I smoked my first tobacco cigarette. Then my second.

It was a night of outward joy and silent, abiding sorrow, like so many before and since.

As the time approached 12 a.m., I could be found standing with my friend in his back garden. There were other pals around us, too — drunkenly yapping and laughing in that loud way inebriated people do. The night was like glass; still, clear. The stars glinted, gazing down on us like thousands of bright, vigilant eyes.

I had consumed several cans of beer and a considerable amount of whiskey.

And I was reminiscing.

'Do you remember when Emma and I did 'Thriller' in Sixth Class?' I slurred.

My friend had stayed sober throughout the evening — he was responsible for the state of the house, and so he had to keep an eye on the rest of us.

He looked at me now, and nodded.

'That song went on a lot longer than you expected,' he stated.

I stared at him. I had never spoken to this friend about my love for Emma. But he knew. Like all my friends who'd read my writing, and who'd heard the way I talked about her, he knew.

There was nothing for me to explain.

After her letter and what I thought was the end of my friendship with Emma, I drank alcohol often. I sipped whiskey on my own, late at night, when my parents and sisters were asleep. My friends bought me the bottles, or I stole from Mai and Des's liquor cabinet. If I knew a pal was coming over, sometimes I would get semi-drunk before he arrived, so I could share my problems more frankly. I needed to talk to whoever would listen. Drinking made it easier.

It wasn't just the Emma situation that was making me hurt.

Because the 'relationship' I had with Emma in Sixth Class was the closest I'd ever come to romance, I guess I placed a lot of faith in friendship. I clung to my friendships; I nurtured them. I didn't hold with the notion that, as events in one's life changed, companionships automatically slipped away.

I usually wasn't the one to phone my friends and ask them if they'd like to meet. I preferred to send emails or the occasional text message — things that could be voluntarily replied to. I didn't like to take up my friends' time with phone calls. But if I requested a friend's help, I expected to get it. Maybe I asked too much of my friends sometimes. But I never asked for anything more than I was prepared to give in return.

In spring 2002, it seemed as if two of my most treasured friendships were dying.

One of these friendships was with an Andrew's pal. After I came out of the HDU, I realised that this friend had become different; whereas before, he and I had been able to share both profound and profoundly wacky conversations, now all we were able to share was small talk. My friend just didn't seem capable of engaging with me anymore, of sharing with me the friendship we'd once shared. I was selfish — I wanted to keep our friendship in aspic; I didn't want it to change. The fact that my friend did change made me bitter and upset for quite a while.

The other of these friendships was with a BSP pal. After my return from the HDU, I texted my BSP pal, to tell him that I'd survived the transplant. This guy had been one of my best friends since I entered First Class. But his reply to my text message consisted of three words: 'Who is this?' He had deleted my number from the phonebook on his mobile. He didn't even know that I'd spent the previous three months in hospital. That, naturally, stabbed at my soul.

Over time, the fissures in both of these friendships would be sealed. Going into the future, I would remain close to my Andrew's pal and my BSP pal.

But in spring 2002, I felt abandoned by two of my oldest and closest companions, as well as by Emma.

Slowly, though, I pulled myself together. My whiskey-sipping became more sporadic. The pools of self-pity dried up; I got on with my schoolwork, and with the magazine.

In May 2002, I compiled a collection of my own writing that contained articles I'd written for *TF*, as well as old English essays, and some new bits and pieces. I photocopied the collection and gave copies to doctors, teachers, relatives, and friends — all the people to whom I owed so much.

One person who received a copy was Emma. The collection was dedicated to her, and several of the reflections therein were veiled commentaries on our turbulent relationship.

Four days after posting Emma's mag, I received a phone call from her.

'Hello?' I said into my mobile.

'I'm a bitch, amn't I?' Emma said.

I feigned ignorance. 'What are you talking about?'

'The collection of writing,' she responded. 'It's fucking amazing. Can I read it to my friends?'

I was taken aback. 'Sure,' I answered, 'I'd be honoured.'

But Emma spoke over my reply. 'I really hurt you, didn't I? I'm so sorry.'

'Well, there were some things you did that caused me pain for a while,' I admitted. 'But then I grew up.' I laughed nervously.

Emma, however, had more to say. From the other end of the line, it sounded like she was taking a deep breath.

'Ben . . . I hope you know,' she began, 'that you made me feel the most loved I ever have been in my life. And I'm so grateful.'

Emma's words sunk into my soul, like stones sinking in water.

'And I hope,' she went on, 'that there isn't any . . . bad feeling, between us anymore.'

How could there be, after a speech like that?

'Not if you promise we'll always be friends,' I replied.

And then I felt guilty. For the first time, I was seeing things from Emma's viewpoint. She had been only fifteen years old when I told her that I was in love with her; to hear those words from a seriously ill friend must have been like a grenade going off in her ear. I knew she must have gone out with other guys since Sixth Class, but I'd never told her that, more than anything, I just wanted to see her happy. I wanted to say how unimaginably sorry I was. But my guilt couldn't find its way into words.

'Thanks for listening,' Emma said. 'Bye.'

Somehow, Emma's apology and my swelling guilt made me want her more than ever.

Early in the summer school term of 2002, I paid another visit to St Andrew's College — ostensibly to meet with teachers, but really just to chat with friends. During this visit, I bumped into my first 'Emma' confidante — that blonde, bubbly, American English teacher. The teacher told me that she was planning on returning to the US for good. She would be leaving once the summer exams passed.

On my next visit to Andrew's, I brought with me a copy of my recently thrown-together collection of writings, and handed it to my former teacher. I'd placed the collection in a sealed envelope, and I'd included in the envelope a letter, filled with details of the latest 'Emma & Ben' developments.

Later that night, I received an email from my one-time English teacher. She wrote that she was sorry to hear that Emma and I had never got together. But she promised that Emma's lack of romantic feelings for me would only bring me closer to my true love, who she knew was out there.

I didn't dare believe her. Hope is an addictive drug. You can't just give it up; but there's so much hurt when it's all you've got.

May sailed into June, and the first anniversary of my bone marrow transplant arrived. My family and I didn't do anything particularly special. We got a Chinese takeaway — it was nice to be able to eat those again!

The last twelve months had overflowed with emotion and turmoil. But things were looking up. I was beavering away at my studies, preparing to head straight into my final year at St Andrew's College. My hospital visits were down to once every three months. Instead of having to take thirty pills a day, I now had to take only one — an antibiotic that I would be on for the rest of my life (even though I'd had a transplant, my immune system was still never going to be fully normal).

On my anniversary, my dad gave me a gift, a book entitled *Poems for Refugees*. He handed me a card with the gift. I opened the card first.

> *Ben,*
> *One year on, it's good to see you healthy and happy again. Well, healthy anyway. We'll continue to work on the happiness.*
> *Forever,*
> *Des'*

15. 'Now you turn around and tell me I'm not Jesus?!'

One outcome of a successful bone marrow transplant is that, afterwards, the recipient's body contains the DNA of two individuals — his own, and the donor's. During one of my post-transplant visits to Our Lady's, a nurse needed to take a sample of my own DNA, and she told me that the best way to get a good sample was to swab the inside of my mouth. Swimming in my blood is someone else's blueprint. It's quite a strange thought. If I ever turn to a life of crime, the ability to leave someone else's DNA at the scene could come in very handy.

I've never met my bone marrow donor; I've only seen news stories about BMT patients who have met theirs. I suppose it's something I'd like to do some day. It would be nice to thank him or her for giving me the rest of my life. I know, however, that meeting one's donor is not always possible. Sometimes there is a total ban on donor meeting recipient. Aengus informed me that this is in case the recipient ever needs a second transplant. Donors should never feel obligated to give their marrow, and bonds of friendship with a recipient might make them feel so.

After surviving my transplant, I felt bitterly guilty. Doctors and nurses used to tell me that it was my 'strong spirit' that saved me, and this made me mad. To me, it was like saying that all those who die during transplant are without strong spirits. Post-BMT, I wasn't 'strong' — I was broken. I wanted to kill myself.

It wasn't just in the days after my release from the HDU, however, that I thought about suicide. I thought about it before then, and I have thought about it since. Notions of death have never been far from my mind.

Sometimes, when I thought about suicide, I really did feel that my life was worthless. I thought it'd be arrogant to assume my death would affect my friends and family. After all, I was such a pathetic excuse for a man — the girl I was in love with wasn't in love with me, and I had a defective body that needed drugs and other people's blood and other people's insides to keep it alive. What could I possibly do that would be of use to anybody?

Other times, when I thought about suicide, I didn't really feel that my life was worthless. I knew I had a loving family and caring friends, and that I had the ability to write and act and entertain people. I just found it so hard to live through the pain. I yearned every single minute for a love that could never be mine, and I hated the fact that I would have to live the rest of my life in a substandard body. How could I wake up in the morning still feeling like this?

I've thought about the method I would use to kill myself, I've written suicide notes, but I've never attempted suicide. In a strange way, I often found my suicidal thoughts comforting. They provided a cushion for all my worries about life. It was a relief to know that if my situation got really, unbearably awful, I could just kill myself and that would be that.

It's also strange to think of the things that would set off my suicidal thoughts. Often, with regard to my illness, it was the little indignities that made me want to leave this body behind just as much as the big challenges. These small things made me realise that, no matter how well I was, my life would always be a little different from my friends'.

In the spring of 2002, I still had to wear a mask while in Our Lady's. Every time I went for a checkup, I had to cover my nose and mouth. This was because there was construction going on around the hospital. During one visit, I was in St John's, getting blood test forms to bring to the phlebotomist (by this time, outpatients' blood samples were no longer taken on the ward—they were all taken by the phlebotomist, who was based down the other end of the hospital). Frieda, the Bone Marrow Transplant Coordinator, handed me my forms, along with a mask.

But I refused to put on the mask. It just seemed like I'd been through enough. I'd had needles jabbed into me for eight years; I'd had tubes shoved into almost every part of my body; I'd suffered physical and mental humiliation throughout my transplant. Now I was supposed to be getting better—I was going to school (albeit sporadically), I felt healthy and strong, my blood counts were normal for the first time in nearly a decade. Yet here I was, being asked to cover my face while walking down a corridor. I couldn't take it anymore.

It was an unforgivably selfish stance. Frieda snatched the mask and the blood forms from my hands, and refused to allow me go anywhere. She then marched off in anger.

After a few minutes, I approached her apologetically. I said I would wear the mask. Frieda smiled and told me that she understood how I felt. She stressed that it was only for my own safety that I had to wear the mask.

I accepted the forms, put on the mask, and walked through the hospital corridors to the phlebotomist. The phlebotomist took some of my blood, and then taped a piece of cotton wool over the little puncture the needle had left in my arm. I said 'Thanks', and went on my way.

That was one of the last times I had to don a mask in public. And hopefully it will be for many years to come.

I would never say that the transplant, my experiences in the HDU, and the experiences of my recovery, didn't change me. Though I'm not really sure how much they changed me. Every year, every day, changes me in some way, I guess, as I absorb new memories, meet new people, write more, read more, and watch more TV and movies. I still think I'm essentially the same person I was before my BMT — even if I do have new DNA.

I suppose, if I'm being honest, I would have to tell you that one of the first things that happened to me personality-wise post-transplant was that I became less tolerant of other people's problems. All my friends' difficulties seemed idiotically trivial compared to mine. This self-absorption, however, soon drained away; I'd like to think that, in the end, the experiences of my transplant helped me to be a better friend, and A Better Ben.

I don't tend to have good and bad days anymore. I still find life hard — I've yet to meet someone who doesn't. But every day seems to have so much in it, so many poems waiting to be found and written. I like the search.

In terms of the physical consequences of the transplant, I am blessed that they have been few. I haven't yet developed graft versus host disease, or any form of cancer. Cataracts have not yet grown on my eyes.

About a year after my transplant, however, I did develop a constant, throbbing pain in my right foot. I met with a physiotherapist, who told me I had probably just sprained my ankle. The pain didn't go away, though. So I went to Our Lady's to have an x-ray. When the doctor showed me the x-ray images, I saw that, around my right ankle, there was a dark grey patch of bone. The rest of my bones on both feet were bright white.

The orthopaedic consultant told me that I had avascular necrosis of the talus. In other words—a problem with the blood supply to a small bone in my ankle. The problem was probably caused by the heavy doses of steroids I'd endured during my BMT, and not helped by the fact that I was on oxymethalone for six and a half years before that. The consultant said the pain was as a result of cartilage being worn down and two bones grating against each other.

'It's relatively common,' the consultant said of avascular necrosis. 'But it's more often found in the hip. If you had it there, we could drill into the bone with a special drill to try and stimulate the blood supply.'

But, because the talus was so small, this procedure couldn't really be attempted on my ankle, the doctor told me. I might end up with irreversible damage to my foot.

'We could get you an artificial ankle,' he went on, 'but I wouldn't recommend that, unless you really start having trouble moving. The way you are now, if you were to get an artificial ankle, you'd end up with less movement, and the same amount of pain. Maybe, if your ankle gets worse, it's something to think about down the road.

'You never know,' the orthopaedic consultant concluded, 'it could get worse or then again it could get better. You just never know.'

This constant, throbbing pain in my ankle hasn't affected my life too much. When I'm just sitting around the house, the pain is unnoticeable. My right foot, however, always feels like it's only half-attached to the rest of my leg. I have to wear a foot brace, and I got orthotics made to put in my shoes. Sometimes, especially when I have to do a lot of walking, the pain does get quite bad, and I'll start limping. I can't really run anymore.

Avascular necrosis wasn't the only problem that emerged about a year post-transplant. Around the same time, I developed an unquenchable thirst. I had this bizarre feeling of always needing a drink. In the morning, after a night without any water, my mouth would be almost painfully dry. No matter how much I drank, however, the thirst wouldn't go away completely.

I was tested for diabetes, and for GVHD — another possibility. Both results, however, came back negative. Dr O'Marcaigh and the Crumlin team were perplexed. What could be causing this thirst?

Over a year would pass before I was given a reason, and offered a solution.

During the summer of 2002, I was finding it quite hard to read. My psychotic episode had shattered my attention span, and I was still trying to put it back together. I'd read three paragraphs, and then have to go back and read them again. My mind would meander off, even as my eyes continued to follow the lines on the page.

Oddly, one of the reasons I was finding it so hard to read was that I kept getting distracted by ideas for my own writing. That summer, I wrote a lot. I had grown to love more than ever the process of trying to sculpt something beautiful, or meaningful, or humorous, from words. I usually wrote longhand at night, often while listening to music. During the day, I'd type up the previous night's musings, editing them at the same time. Most of the pieces I was penning were for *Totally Fushed*.

Since the first issue in 2000, *TF* had only grown bigger and better. Loads of my friends were now writing for it, as were people I knew through the Internet and people I didn't know at all. We were getting new readers all the time.

Over the years, the mag had allowed me to create my own reality. Or escape from reality — the reality of my illness. Some of the stories I wrote and printed in *TF*, such as the one about the boy who bullied sheep by reading poems to them, or the one about the alien who was attacked by a serial killer on a beach — these were a world away from lying on a hospital bed, depending on blood transfusions for life.

And yet, *Totally Fushed* was vitally near to this aspect of my life, too. I'd needed my mag through the years. Without it, I would never have known where to turn for comfort.

In the summer of '02, I wrote the first short story based on my transplant for *TF*. In many ways, the story was a dry run for this book. The subplot involved my hero's feelings for a girl he fell in love with when he was twelve. I also began avidly scribbling poetry for the first time that summer (previously I'd only dabbled in the craft).

New writing opportunities were presenting themselves, as well. I'd always liked writing about the interesting things that happened in my life. And in summer '02, something very interesting happened. I got to act in *Fair City*!

Okay, well, 'act' is a bit extreme.

I got to walk behind some tables in *Fair City*!

My uncle Gerard is one of the stars of the RTÉ soap opera, and the producers of the show had been looking for a homeless person, so, of course, my name came to Gerard's mind, and he passed it on to his employers.

I had an interesting day at the Dundrum Community Centre, which was serving as a homeless shelter. I learned how little of TV acting is actually about the actors. There is waiting, and deciding on angles, and editing and directing, and moving props and installing wiring and takes and retakes and constant clouds of smoke and sputtering as cigarettes are sucked like they're about to be banned . . . I swear, every time there was a break in filming, every person present would light up. If I ever land a job in TV, before I take it up, I'll have to become a chain smoker.

After I'd filmed my tone-raising, verisimilitudinous, walking-behind-the-tables cameo, courtesy of a request from Gerard, I got to sit with the director of that particular *Fair City* episode. That was fun, too—to see the process involved in directing the show, to see how the director interacts with the cameramen and the rest of the crew.

Overall, it was a good day. I came away knowing that my parents and friends would get to see me on TV in a few weeks' time. Plus, I got an exclusive for *TF*. And I received my first pay cheque for an acting job.

When I got home after my morning and afternoon as a soap opera extra, I began to write about it right away. Writing about my life had become an essential part of living it. I now knew that, whatever career path I took, I would want it to leave room for my writing.

When I returned fulltime to St Andrew's in August 2002, I began considering college options, and writing and acting were naturally the interests that were foremost in my mind. I thought about studying English at university level. But it seemed that English at the major Irish universities tended to focus on critiquing great literary works rather than on creative writing. And, egoist that I was, I'd always been far more interested in developing my own creativity than commenting on that of others.

I considered many other college courses during the autumn/winter term of 2002: Politics, Philosophy, History, Journalism, even Law. As a kid, in spite of the fact that writing and acting were activities I indulged in constantly, I'd never wanted to be a professional writer or a professional actor. I wanted to become a scientist, or an engineer who designed environmentally friendly cars. Unfortunately, I had no aptitude for science or for engineering — but hey, a kid can dream!

Now, though, acting and writing seemed like the only viable career paths — the only things I was interested enough in and good enough at to pursue. I knew that, whatever direction I went in, I would keep writing — my writing wasn't dependant on having a college course to support it. So, what I was left with was my addiction to the stage. I needed to pursue this addiction, even if it never took me very far.

I spoke to the St Andrew's guidance counsellor about Drama courses. She told me that Trinity College Dublin offered two of the best in the country. One of these, Drama and Theatre Studies, was an Arts degree course. It was an academic course that covered all aspects of theatre, providing many practical classes along the way, including in acting. Trinity accepted just fifteen or so people to Drama and Theatre Studies every year, and admission was based on Leaving Cert points and an interview at the college. The points requirement was quite high. For the previous few years, it had been around five hundred.

The second TCD course that the guidance counsellor told me about was the Bachelor in Acting Studies — the only degree-level actor training programme in Ireland. This was a demanding practical acting course, which focused on making master thespians of its students. You could not apply for the BAS through the usual channel of the Central Applications Office, but had to apply directly to Trinity. This was because entry was not based on Leaving Certificate points at all, but solely on one's performance at an audition. Only about a dozen people got into the course each year.

I applied for a Drama and Theatre Studies place, and for a Bachelor in Acting Studies place. I received two elaborate application forms, which required me to detail my acting experience, to critique some plays I had recently seen, and to list any talents/interests I had besides drama. I really had to sell myself when filling out the forms, as not everyone who filled them out would be called for interview/audition. I was uncomfortable with some of this self-selling. It just felt very egomaniacal. I mean, sure, I had a colossal ego, but I was used to masking it with self-deprecating wit.

Despite my misgivings, I completed both forms, and popped them in the post. Now all I could do was hope that Trinity would buy the stuff I was selling.

Even in those early days of Sixth Year, I was pretty busy with class work and homework, as well as my new duties as a prefect. In some subjects, I still had large sections of the Fifth Year course to cover. I would obviously have to do this on my own. I didn't think I'd have time for any extracurricular activities.

In November '02, however, auditions for the 2003 One-Act Drama Festival were held. Eight schools would be competing. Kristian Marken would be reprising his role as director of the Andrew's production. The play Mr Marken had decided to direct was John Godber's *Teechers*—a comedy set in an English comprehensive school.

In the past, auditions for the One-Act had been open only to Fourth and Fifth Years. This time around, however, because of low turnout among those years, Sixth Years were allowed to audition as well.

Despite this seemingly fateful twist of events, I initially told myself that the Leaving Cert was my total priority, and that I shouldn't go dallying in after-school enjoyment.

But when a friend who'd been involved in the 2002 One-Act asked me if I was going to audition, I suddenly found that I couldn't resist.

I waited outside the St Andrew's main hall during lunch break on one of the audition days. I stood a little way away from a gaggle of yapping girls, who also seemed to be waiting to audition. A shortish, stocky, trim-bearded man approached us. He looked at me.

'One-Act auditions?' he said.

I nodded. This was obviously Kristian.

Kristian led the girls, one other guy, and me to a classroom. There, we read aloud extracts from *Teechers*. When the auditions were over, Kristian thanked us, and told us that a cast list would soon be posted on one of the school's notice boards.

A couple of days later, I checked the notice board. I'd been given the role of Mr Basford, the fascistic school vice-principal. I was going to act again!

We started rehearsals for *Teechers* soon after the auditions. There were fifteen other people in the cast, and I had fabulous fun working with them and with Kristian. Mr Marken was eager to spice up our production with all manner of wacky additions, including cheese-throwing ninjas and flying rubber chickens!

Christmas passed, the new year began, and we continued to rehearse *Teechers*. It no longer seemed appropriate, however, to term our production 'Teechers by John Godber'. In the programme for the One-Act Festival, we should have relabelled it 'John Godber's *Teechers* as adapted and rewritten by Kristian Marken and his cast'. Not as pithy, I know — but it would've been more accurate. To start with, Kristian had to chop out numerous scenes in order to turn the original two-act *Teechers* into a forty-five-minute one-act play. Then, as each rehearsal went by, more and more St Andrew's College in-jokes were added to the dialogue.

One afternoon, we were rehearsing on the stage in the main hall. We were practising a scene in which Mr Basford bursts into the classroom of the school's new Drama teacher, Mr Nixon. Mr Nixon and his students have been making a lot of noise, and Mr Basford is upset about this.

'I can't hear myself think!' the vice-principal screeches.

As the scene unfolds, Mr Basford grows increasingly apoplectic, until he is nose-to-nose with Nixon, screaming — barely coherently — into the Drama teacher's face.

Kristian thought it would be an hilarious idea to change my lines slightly. He wanted me to become so insane with rage that, by the time I reached Nixon, all I was able to come out with was the completely meaningless phrase, 'not one finger'.

I performed the scene as Kristian had asked. I shouted at Nixon, and then, after Nixon made an insolent comment, I inched toward the Drama teacher, my finger outstretched, my eyes bulging, the rage swelling and swelling inside me. I felt the lines weave their way into my blood; I was more alive than I had been at any time since my last One-Act performance. I had this energy, this literal energy that I could feel vibrating in my fingertips. I could do anything — to my own emotions, or to the emotions of my audience.

I got face-to-face with Nixon. Mr Basford was quivering, grasping for words to express his wrath. 'NOT-ONE-FINGER!' I spluttered.

Then Mr Basford spun around, and let out a shriek of utter frustration and fury, before thundering out of the classroom.

When I walked back onto the stage several seconds later, my co-stars were all staring at me.

'Ben can act!' one remarked.

I glanced at the floor.

'That was so brilliant, Ben,' Kristian praised. 'But . . .' He suggested how I could squeeze even more from the scene.

We ran through the scene again, and I tried to do as he'd recommended.

When we'd finished, Kristian joked, 'And the Best Actor goes to . . .'

I smiled, and we moved on to rehearsing another part of the play.

Two days before the night of our One-Act performance, I came down with the flu and a severe fever. Twenty-four hours before I was due to star in *Teechers*, I had pains everywhere; I had unstoppable shivers, a temperature of forty-one degrees Celsius, and my voice was waning.

I took a lot of medication, and went to bed early.

The following morning, I didn't feel much better. But the shakes had stopped, my fever had gone down a little, and with Olbas pastilles and cough syrup, my nose and throat stayed clear.

I went into school. I wasn't going to be left behind. And I couldn't let my friends and co-stars down, no matter how sick I felt.

That afternoon, we ran through *Teechers* for the final time. I tried not to overdo my lines, wary of wearing out my voice.

Once our last rehearsal was over, I took the DART to my dad's office, and met my parents and sisters for a Chinese meal in a nearby restaurant.

After the meal, I returned to Booterstown. I stepped off the train, and spotted Emma and Michelle strolling out of the station. They were on their way up to Andrew's to watch the play. I started to follow them.

It was dark now. As I walked, mizzle from the dismal, black sky caressed my face.

I was feeling a little impish, so I strolled passed the two girls, pretending I hadn't noticed them.

'Ben?' Michelle called from behind me.

I turned around to my two friends, one of whom was the girl who still invaded my dreams.

I smiled.

'Didn't you see us?' Emma inquired.

'No,' I lied. 'I didn't know it was you.'

We crossed the road under the orange light of the streetlamps. As we headed up Booterstown Avenue, I chatted to the twins about *Teechers*. When we got to the school, I showed the girls around St Andrew's.

After the tour, the twins went to buy tickets for the performance. This was the concluding night of the festival. Our play was due to be performed first, but the twins' tickets would also entitle them to stay for the second play, and for the festival's awards ceremony.

I stood in the queue with Emma and Michelle for a few minutes. It was terrific to see a few of my other friends, and some of my relations, arriving. Gerard was there, as was John Douglas, the man who had helped me with the Fifth Year English course after my transplant.

After a short while, I left Emma and Michelle, and went to my locker. I gulped down some cough syrup, swallowed two Panadol tablets, and then popped an Olbas pastille into my gob.

Even though I'd finished a meal only an hour before, I was ravenous. This probably had something to do with the fact that, on account of sickness, I'd eaten very little over the previous two days.

I wasn't able to sort out my hunger just at that moment, however.

I shut my locker, and joined the rest of the *Teechers* cast in our classroom qua dressing room. It was time for me to put on Mr Basford's green suit, and to get my makeup applied.

At 7.30 p.m., the rest of the cast and I made our way to our 'first positions'.

Our production of *Teechers* did not begin on the stage, but in the audience.

Once the lights went down, we stood up and started shouting at one another. Then we all barged through the audience, and marched onto the stage.

In my first proper scene, Mr Basford stormed into the headmistress's office, slammed his hand down on the table (ouch!), and demanded to know why he hadn't been given the lead role in the school's production of *Jesus Christ Superstar*.

'After all the work I put in, now you turn around and tell me I'm not Jesus?' I screamed. 'Great!'

Shortly after this, Mr Basford strutted into his classroom, immediately silencing his hitherto gossiping pupils. Each pupil raised his or her right arm, giving a fascist salute.

I hailed my own brilliance as a Maths teacher. 'I am a genius,' I told the assembled spectators.

It was a fun part to play!

The rest of the production went exceptionally well — the audience seemed to love it. I even got unprompted applause following my 'not one finger' scene!

After our performance, there was a short interval before the next play. Once my co-stars and I had all hugged and congratulated each other, I strolled out of the main hall, still wearing Mr Basford's suit. Along the way, I accepted shouts of 'Well done!' and shook the hands of students from my school and other schools.

I looked around for Emma and Michelle, but they had already headed home.

As I walked through the blue double doors at the back of the hall, however, I spotted someone else I'd want to talk to — Mr Malachi Friel. I hadn't seen my one-time drama teacher since Transition Year.

I went over to him and smiled. 'I didn't know if I'd ever see you again, sir,' I said.

Mr Friel smiled back. 'I didn't know if I'd ever see you again, Ben — if you know what I mean.'

Unfortunately, Mr Friel had just arrived, so he hadn't witnessed *Teechers*. Nevertheless, he and I discussed the forthcoming awards presentation. 'I always found it hard to get the top awards,' he commented, referring to the Big Four — Best Actor, Best Actress, Best Director, and Best Production.

As Mr Friel and I chatted, one of the three St Andrew's vice-principals approached us. The vice-principal greeted Mr Friel and me, and then the two teachers got talking. I slipped off to the school canteen, where refreshments were being served.

I was beginning to feel quite unwell. I was coming down from the high of the performance, and my flu was kicking in again. My face was clammy. I was weak, and still very hungry.

Soon, a bell sounded, and everybody flocked to the St Andrew's main hall once again. The evening's second play commenced.

After the curtain had come down on Mount Temple Comprehensive School's production of *Over the Wall* by James Saunders, the festival's two judges climbed onto the stage to offer their comments on the night's theatre. 'I don't know about a genius of a Maths teacher,' said one of them, 'but certainly a genius of an actor.'

Members of the audience whooped and clapped. And beneath my sickly sweat, I'm sure I blushed just a little.

Following their comments, there was another brief intermission, while the judges deliberated over the presentation of awards.

By now, I had a thumping headache. It was hard to stand up. My throat was aching.

Nonetheless, when that bell rang out, signalling that the adjudicators had reached their decisions, I returned to the hall for the awards ceremony. I was one of the last to enter the hall, however. By the time I arrived, all the seats were taken. I stood at the back, leaning against a metal bar.

The first accolades to be handed out were the Certificates of Merit. One member of our troupe was given a certificate for her portrayal of a student who tries to seduce Mr Nixon. I was delighted for her, because she really had been superb.

After the Runner-Up Best Actress award and the Best Actress award had been presented, the adjudicators read out the name of the Runner-Up Best Actor.

It wasn't me.

Then: 'And the winner of the 2003 Best Actor award . . . Ben Murnane, St Andrew's College, for Mr Basford in *Teechers*!'

The audience's silence exploded into cheers and applause.

My mind did a backflip. Happiness crashed down on top of me . . . but I was so weak, I thought I was going to faint! I took my hands off the metal railing, and moved up the hall. Several of my co-stars were sitting just in front of the stage. When I reached them, they put their arms around me and called me a 'legend'.

My feet felt heavy and my head felt unbearably light as I climbed onto the stage. It took all of my focus just to navigate the steps but I did it.

The Headmaster presented me with the perpetual Best Actor cup. 'Congratulations, Ben,' he said over the continuing noise.

'Thank you, sir,' I managed, grinning and shaking his hand.

'Wait,' he said, 'you're not finished yet.' He then gave me my replica trophy, which I would be allowed to keep forever.

I made it down off the stage. But I only stayed off for a few moments.

After Runner-Up Best Production had been awarded, one of the adjudicators said, smiling, 'And we can present the next two awards together.'

Teechers won Best Production, and Kristian won Best Director. The crowd — saturated with Andrew's students — hollered, whistled, and clapped. And I climbed back onto the stage, this time with all of my co-stars and with Kristian. It was a moment brimming with magic.

Adrenaline had obviously started pumping, because suddenly my hunger and my headache faded — strength burst into my limbs.

I found my parents and sisters and hugged them.

I laughed with my co-stars. We posed for a photo for the school magazine. The grinning and the celebrating didn't stop until we parted, and even then it continued — we just didn't do it together!

At about 11 p.m., Mai, Des, Ruth, Jess, and I left St Andrew's through the twin sets of double doors that formed the main entrance to the school. When I reached the cool outside air, I drank in the night. The stars stuck out in the sky like bubbles in champagne.

As we walked toward the car, one of the festival adjudicators strode past me.

I thanked him for the Best Actor award.

The adjudicator spun around to face me, and smiled.

'It wasn't even close,' he said.

16. Tennis balls

The following chill morning, after a night during which gloating phone calls were made to grandparents and faraway friends, I stood on Platform 1 at Bray DART Station. I was waiting for the 7.55 train. A friend who had also been in *Teechers* was with me.

I turned to him. 'Aren't we legends?' I said.

My pal squinted at me through sleepy eyes, and grinned. 'Are you coming to the party tonight?' he asked.

'Yep,' I confirmed. A cast party was being held that evening at the house of one of our co-stars. This party was not exclusively for the *Teechers* cast, however. Earlier in the week, St Andrew's students had put on a production of Peter Weiss's *Marat/Sade*, and a production of *Riders to the Sea* by J. M. Synge. The students who worked on these two shows were invited to our co-star's party as well.

I didn't like attending parties at which there would be lots of people I didn't know. My self-confidence always scuttled away; I became quiet and shy, and I tended to spend a lot of time in corners. I'd searched for an excuse to get out of going to our co-star's party — but I really didn't have one.

So, some twelve hours later, my DARTing friend and I arrived at our co-star's house. We were among the first guests to turn up. Pretty soon, though, droves of Fourth, Fifth, and Sixth Years began pouring in. I tried to fade into the furniture. This didn't work, however. I had won Best Actor, and everyone wanted to congratulate me.

An hour or so after the party started, I wandered into the living room. Camcorder footage of our *Teechers* performance was playing on the TV. I just caught the end of my 'not one finger' scene.

A lad I didn't know was standing in front of the television. He leaned over to the girl beside him, and said, 'He's brilliant, isn't he?'

'He's standing right behind you,' she replied.

The guy turned, saw me, and chuckled. 'It would've been funnier if we were saying you were crap!' he commented.

'Yes,' I agreed, laughing.

Before the cast party had begun, I'd decided I wasn't going to drink that night. When a friend popped open a bottle of champagne, however, I couldn't resist. I ended up drinking half the damn thing. Then I stood drunkenly in the kitchen, gazing in both admiration and amusement at my fellow teenagers, who were happily dancing to music blaring from a stereo in the corner.

There was only one other person in the room who wasn't dancing — a slim girl, slightly shorter than me, with long, straight brown hair, and glasses. The girl noticed me, and came over to where I was standing. I knew her name was Aisling. She was in the year below mine, and was friendly with some of my pals. On occasion, Aisling had taken the train to school with us in the morning. But I'd never spoken to her, beyond exchanging bland pleasantries.

Aisling had been heavily involved in the music for the *Marat/Sade*. I knew how talented a musician she was — I'd seen her play the piano and the flute at school assemblies. I also knew of her gift for art — I'd seen some of her work in the St Andrew's creative journal, *The Wine Dark Sea*.

Aisling congratulated me on my performance and my award.

She smiled playfully. 'Can you do something from *Teechers* for me here now?' she asked.

I was drunk enough to be happy to oblige.

I moved a few feet away from Aisling, and turned my back to her. Then I spun around. I moved haltingly towards her, as if each step were making me madder and madder. I reached Aisling. 'NOT-ONE-FINGER!' I yelled.

The people surrounding us clapped, and Aisling thanked me.

Aisling wasn't drinking alcohol. She said she didn't need to, as she could simulate being drunk by twirling in circles. She started to spin herself around, and encouraged me to join in. I tried her trick, but, since I was already 'under the influence', I just began to feel utterly dazed, nauseous, and without balance. I had to lean against a countertop for support.

As the dancers grew weary and the kitchen became empty, Aisling and I moved to the crowded sitting room. I confessed my desire to sit down.

'You can have half a seat,' Aisling said, and we shared an armchair.

As I finished my last glass of champagne, I got up to sneak a Heineken from the fridge.

When I returned to her, however, Aisling wouldn't let me drink my Heineken from the can. She thought I'd had enough alcohol, so she rationed the beer into my champagne glass as she saw fit.

We laughed, we talked; I was relaxed and cheerful for the first time in ages. I felt like an explorer who'd just discovered something astonishing.

After the One-Act had passed, the Leaving Cert could again be given my full attention. I was enjoying my classes in school, particularly English. We were covering some of my favourite poets — Robert Frost, Derek Mahon, Sylvia Plath.

When the 2003 Easter holidays arrived, however, I had no time for leisure. Over the Easter break, as well as revising my Sixth Year notes, I continued to work on vast sections of the Fifth Year course that I'd either completely forgotten or never covered. Having to do all this extra work with only a few months to go till the exams naturally dumped more pressure on me. But, for some reason, I wasn't feeling unbearably stressed.

I was amazed at my own attitude, actually, considering what I'd been like in the run-up to my Junior Cert. I wasn't putting in any less effort now than I had then; if anything, I was studying even more. But I no longer worried so much about the work, about getting good grades. I still wanted to do the best I could — and I knew I would do the best I could. I just wasn't going to fry my mind thinking about the exams. Two years before, I'd nearly died. The Leaving Cert could move down my list of priorities.

It was interesting how my classmates' attitudes to exams had evolved over the years, as well. I guess most of them moved in the opposite direction to me. They went from not caring about school-work to viewing the Leaving Cert as the ultimate determinant of their future lives. In First Year, if you were top of the class, you were mocked by your fellow pupils. In Sixth Year, they looked up to you as an example. Childlike attitudes — to school, at any rate — had slipped away over the half-dozen years. I'd always studied, but I'd always kept secret the amount of studying I actually did. Now, all of a sudden, studying was what everyone wanted to be able to do. Nerds could reveal themselves to the world.

As the Easter holidays became memories and my final term in secondary school began, I continued to fill as many hours as I could with study.

It's quite a lonely activity, really. I'd never been much good at learning in 'group study' sessions, or even in class. I needed to be on my own with a textbook, a pad of paper, and a pen—and I'd just write things over and over until they were sufficiently rammed into my head.

I was less stressed than I was before my Junior Cert, but I was finding study harder than I'd found it previously. The reading was difficult, because of the post-BMT attention-span trouble that was still with me. Often, while studying, I'd get frustrated, and end up staring into the distance for minutes on end, thinking about the things that happened to me during the transplant, or about Emma.

I still loved her so much.

I needed to speak to someone about Emma, face to face. I needed to be able to just talk—to explore out loud how I felt and hopefully come away understanding my own emotions better. I'd long ago accepted that Emma was not going to fall in love with me. But I was still looking for a way to move on.

I realised that I had a psychologist, a person who'd been through my bone marrow transplant with me and seen some of my darkest hours—Dr Gina MacDonnell.

I tried to get in touch with Gina in May 2003. I didn't know if she would be able to help me, but I wanted to at least make an effort to calm my feelings for Emma before the start of the Leaving Cert. I didn't want to be distracted during my exams.

But Gina was away, or sick, or something. I wasn't able to see her before the Leaving Cert began.

Once 2003's Easter holidays had turned into 2003's summer school term, the end of our second-level educational careers loomed over my head and my friends' heads like a colossal question mark. None of us knew where we were going to be after the Leaving Cert. Our teachers told us to suspend our social lives for the next few months, and most of us were happy to do so. Nobody wanted to end up not getting enough points and having to repeat the year.

One morning, during our class's roll call, with all my classmates listening, my form teacher asked me to give a speech during my year's last ever assembly at St Andrew's College. Each of the year's six forms was supposed to have someone speak at the assembly.

All my classmates turned to look at me as our teacher made the request.

'Um, I don't think so,' I said, trying to display a sort of trendy lack of interest.

'Ah, you will,' our teacher replied.

And that, it seemed, was the end of the matter.

But I didn't mind. In truth, I was excited about giving the speech. It would be an opportunity to entertain my schoolmates, and to get up on the Andrew's stage again.

I had about a week to craft my talk. It only had to be two or three minutes long, and humour, naturally, was the order of the day. I put in one or two funny anecdotes, but the speech still seemed quite serious.

So, on the morning of Final Assembly, when I got up in front of all the Fifth and Sixth Years to give the speech, I spoke in a sarcastic tone. Nobody thought the speech was serious then. I stood behind the blue, crest-emblazoned pulpit from which the Headmaster usually made his weekly announcements. My audience, my schoolmates, were in a party mood. And I wanted to do justice to the occasion. This wasn't any run-of-the-mill speech, after all. Aisling and all my other Andrew's friends were watching.

I closed by saying, 'And now we're only left with the small matter of the Leaving Certificate. But, having attended the prestigious St Andrew's College, what could possibly go wrong?'

A few weeks later, our year's Valedictory Night was held.

My schoolmates and I didn't have to wear our uniforms on Valedictory Night, but we did have to be in formal get-up. The boys wore suits and the girls wore dresses. I didn't know which was more momentous — that my days at St Andrew's College were coming to an end, or that I was wearing for the first time a suit of my own. My parents had bought me a dashing, navy, Marks & Spencer two-piece for the occasion.

After the Valedictory Night speeches, and after a stand-up meal of beef and rice, all the other members of my year and I made our way to Monkstown Rugby Club. We had hired a bar, and it was time to get drunk.

A few hours and several drinks into the evening, I went to the toilet. As I stood at the sink, washing my hands, one of my friends walked in. Then another guy walked in—a tall lad. I didn't know this second guy that well; I hadn't spoken to him much over the years.

The tall guy looked at my friend and me, and said, drunkenly, 'You two better fucking sign my yearbook. I'll fucking cry if you don't.'

I made sure to sign his yearbook before the night was over.

Obviously, that night was an emotional one. We would never be together as a year again, except during the Leaving Cert—and that didn't really count. I was happy being drunk in the smoky, loud-with-music darkness. But I did also feel a certain sadness. I'd spent five years going to the same classes as these people, and I knew hardly any of them.

As we left the rugby club, I exchanged farewell cheek kisses with girls to whom I had never chatted before, and promised lads with whom I was similarly unacquainted that I would go for drinks with them soon.

It was a night full of goodbyes with which nothing was lost, and full of promises that would never be kept.

Two days before my Leaving Certificate exams began with English Papers 1 and 2, I got a letter informing me that my Trinity Bachelor in Acting Studies audition would be held on 9 July 2003.

Some weeks before, I'd been called for a Drama and Theatre Studies interview. I was chuffed to get the call because, as I later found out, only a third of the people who'd applied for Drama and Theatre places actually wound up with interviews. Shortly after mine, I received a letter confirming that I had passed it. Now all I needed to qualify for Drama and Theatre Studies were the considerable Leaving Cert points.

With the DTS interview out of the way, my attention could turn to the BAS audition—once I was finished my Leaving Cert.

The day after I got the missive about my audition, I was sitting on my bed, my head buried in English notes. There was a knock on my door, and my mum entered the room.

'Mr Agnew's on the phone for you,' she announced.

I went to the phone.

'Hello?' I said.

Mr Agnew told me he was just ringing to thank me for the presents.

On my last day of lessons in St Andrew's, I'd given several of my teachers gifts. As I didn't have direct access to Mr Agnew (what with him not teaching anymore), I'd given my History teacher a little bag to pass on to the ex-English teacher. The bag contained a mug, a book token, and a copy of my newest photocopied collection of writings.

Mr Agnew apologised for not having contacted me sooner. He had been very busy, he said. So busy, in fact, that he was redefining his understanding of the word 'priority'.

'I'm not sure I deserve them,' Mr A said of my gifts.

I assured him that he did.

He and I then discussed my writing. Mr Agnew asked me where the creative drive came from. He said that he had never felt the urge to write, though he had on occasion been required to pen speeches and the like for the school.

I said I didn't know why, but I'd just always needed to scribble things—poems, reflections, articles. I told him that the stuff in the collection I'd given him had been written over the previous year or so.

'It seems to be pretty evenly divided between poetry and prose at the moment,' he observed.

'Yeah,' I confirmed. 'I don't know about the poetry, though,' I admitted. I was frustrated with the verse I was writing. I didn't seem able to capture in my poems the emotions I wanted to.

Mr Agnew told me to keep trying. And he passed on a quote he'd once read, about how the way to know a good poem, is to know that it could only have been written by one person. It's the author's own self that gives life to his poetry.

Mr Agnew recognised, however, that writing poems was hard, that it demanded discipline.

'It's about those nights when you're lying awake trying to think of a single phrase,' he said. 'Or a single word, even.'

And he assured me that finding weaknesses in my writing ability was not necessarily a bad thing.

'Yes,' I replied. 'You have to know your limits.'

'Well, not just for that reason. Knowing your weaknesses allows you to focus on your strengths.'

There was one curious thing about my conversation with Mr Agnew on that summer 2003 afternoon. It was the day before Leaving Cert English Papers 1 and 2—and he did not mention my impending exams!

That night, after much study, I went to bed at 2 a.m. I awoke again at 5 a.m. to do more study. This was a pattern I repeated throughout the exam period.

English Papers 1 and 2 were held on Wednesday 4 June, 2003. Both went well. Paper 1 even included a question that gave me an opportunity to write about my transplant.

The remainder of my LC exams also passed without trouble or strife. Once they got started, I slipped into 'exam mode', and it rocket-boosted me through to the end. It was a hectic two weeks, but I wasn't disappointed with any of the papers, unlike some of my classmates. A lot of people didn't like Biology. After that exam, I saw one girl complaining about the paper to a few other students.

'What did you think of it, Ben?' this girl asked as I passed her.

'I thought it was okay,' I said.

'Fuck you!' the girl shouted, and stormed off, muttering to herself.

On Wednesday 18 June, my Leaving Cert ended.

'Now, would you finish up, please,' the invigilator said, as the clock reached 5 p.m.

When everyone's answer booklets had been collected, the invigilator announced, 'You may go.'

I strolled up to one of my friends, and we talked about the paper, before wondering what we should do to celebrate.

It was nearly two years since my bone marrow transplant. And I could see a future falling into place.

For my Bachelor in Acting Studies audition, I had to perform two monologues—one Shakespearean, and one modern (post-1960). The Shakespearean monologue I prepared was from *Macbeth*; the modern piece I prepared was from *The Norman Conquests* by Alan Ayckbourn.

A couple of days before my audition, my uncle Gerard came to Kilmac, and I went through my monologues with him. He got me to try a few useful exercises — for example, reciting a monologue while sitting on my hands! This forced me to focus solely on my voice, on how I was saying the piece.

The *Macbeth* soliloquy I memorised was the one in which Macbeth debates whether or not to murder King Duncan. The first time I performed the piece for Gerard, however, my uncle informed me that it sounded more like I was debating what to have for dinner.

That put me in my place! Gerard suggested that I perform the monologue while standing behind a chair. He suggested that I stand as regally as I could, and that I place my hands on the back of the chair. Gerard figured this stance would prevent me from making any un-kingly movements.

We worked hard and, by the end of our session, Gerard seemed to think I was playing the part much better.

I'd never really thought of acting as 'work' before — it was always just something I 'did'. I'd never really consciously thought about how to play a part — parts always just 'happened' as I read scripts and got a feel for characters.

Gerard taught me a lot that afternoon. And, as he was teaching me, I realised that I still had so much to learn. And I wanted to learn.

Even though I'd also applied for a Drama and Theatre Studies place, a place among the Bachelors in Acting Studies was what I really desired. The BAS was an acting course, not a theatre course. I was much more interested in learning to become an actor than in studying theatre.

On the morning of 9 July, I travelled to Trinity College by DART.

I was nervous. This audition would decide at least some things about my future.

But I was also confident. Even if I had a lot to learn, I was a good actor. I would try my best.

Along with the letter from Trinity telling me about my audition, I was sent a map of the college. The letter instructed me to go to the Samuel Beckett Centre. On the day of my audition, I managed to follow my map to the wrong end of the campus.

I'd walked through the TCD grounds before, but I was now seeing them in a new light. I could end up here pretty soon, I thought. Trinity had grey buildings and redbrick buildings, modern buildings and old buildings, trim green lawns and smooth tarmac pathways.

The most striking feature of the campus, though, for me, was the cherry blossom trees, which were bursting with petals. There was a light breeze that day, and petals were swirling from the trees and falling onto the tarmac pathways like pink, summertime snow.

When I eventually found the Samuel Beckett Centre, I entered its foyer. Adorning the walls were many framed, black and white photographs of Mr Beckett. The ticket desk for the Samuel Beckett Theatre was directly ahead of me as I sauntered through the door.

As I sat in the SBC foyer that morning, I was given an insight into just how coveted BAS places actually were. This was only one of many audition dates, and there were two dozen or so applicants in attendance, ranging in age from my age to middle age. For some, this was their third year applying for a place. Year on year, they kept coming back.

After a short wait, a Drama lecturer arrived to greet my fellow applicants and me. She introduced herself as Chrissie Poulter. Chrissie was middle-aged; she had long, wavy, flaxen hair, and was wearing a navy fleece and brown sandals. She took us into the Samuel Beckett Theatre, and gave us a brief pep talk.

'Today is as much about finding out whether this course is right for you as whether you are right for this course,' she declared.

After Chrissie's short speech, we got stuck into a 'warm-up/get-to-know-your-fellow-applicants' session, which involved such tasks as bouncing imaginary balloons around the room. Typical drama stuff.

Once the session in the Beckett Theatre was over, Chrissie marched us back to the SBC foyer. And then, one by one, we were summoned to perform our monologues in front of three instructors affiliated with the BAS course. These auditions were held in one of the Drama Department's rehearsal studios.

While I waited to be called for my audition, I watched some of the other course-applicants rehearse their pieces. A couple of people were standing on the concrete patio outside the foyer, gesturing and mouthing lines to themselves. I sat at a table inside, occasionally glancing out the window at them. It was obvious how much they all wanted places on this course. I may not have been out there with them, but I still wanted a place as much as anyone.

Eventually, my turn to audition came.

'Hello, Ben,' said Chrissie. She had my BAS application form in her hands. She and the two other instructors were seated at a table at the far end of the room. They seemed a very long way away.

'Hello,' I replied.

I told the three instructors that I would be performing a piece from *Macbeth* and a piece from *The Norman Conquests* by Alan Ayckbourn.

'Do you mind if I use a chair?' I asked.

'No, go ahead,' Chrissie responded. 'Whatever you need.'

I took a brown plastic chair from a stack by the wall, and then returned to the centre of the room.

'Should I just . . . ?' I began.

'Yes. Whenever you're ready,' smiled Chrissie.

And so I stood behind my chair, cleared my throat, and began my *Macbeth* monologue.

Being in that rehearsal room wasn't the same as being onstage. I generally found that the more people there were watching me, the more energy I had to work with in my performance! But I still got a thrill from performing that day.

After I'd uttered the last line of the *Macbeth* piece, I paused for a moment. Then I moved around to the front of the chair, and sat down. I took in a breath, then began the Ayckbourn monologue.

Once my *Norman Conquests* character had finished yelling, I got up from my chair, and placed it back at the side of the room.

'And you also run your own magazine?' Chrissie said, glancing at my application form.

'Yes,' I replied.

'What do you call it?' Chrissie asked.

I smiled. '*Totally Fushed.*'

'I see . . . Well, thank you.'

'Thanks,' I said, and looked at the instructors once more, before leaving the room.

As I walked out the door, the inevitable niggling doubts kicked in. Should I have glanced that way that time? Should I have uttered that line differently?

I had to cast these doubts aside — I'd know soon enough whether my performance had been adequate.

Once we'd performed our monologues, course-applicants were allowed to go for lunch. We were informed that a list of names would be posted on the window of the SBC foyer by 2.30 p.m. Only the people whose names were on this list would be progressing to the next round of the audition process.

I moseyed off to Grafton Street to grab some food, and returned to the SB Centre at about twenty past two.

I stood outside the foyer, waiting with a few other applicants.

After a few minutes, one of my fellow auditionees said to me, 'So, how did you feel when you saw your name on the list?'

'What?' I replied. 'I was just waiting for the list to be put up.'

'But, it's already there,' the auditionee said, pointing toward the window of the foyer.

'Oh.'

What an idiot I was—I hadn't checked the window since returning to the SBC!

There was an awkward pause. The people I'd been waiting with were all advancing to the next round. They had been assuming that I was cleared to go forward as well. It would be pretty embarrassing if my name wasn't actually on the list.

'I—I think I saw your name up there,' the auditionee to whom I'd been talking said.

I walked over to the foyer window, my heart somewhere between my head and my throat. I scanned the list of names.

I turned around to the other applicants, who were looking at me expectantly.

I smiled. 'Yeah, it's there,' I said, as my heart dropped into my chest again.

I had made it through Round One. But none of us standing outside the SBC that afternoon was anywhere near a place on the course yet. The next round was a session of 'movement', to be held shortly.

More than twenty people had turned up for their BAS auditions that morning—but only eight names were on the list on the foyer window. I was glad, of course, that I was one of the applicants who'd been called back. But my heart bled as I watched others arrive, gaze hopefully at the list, and then walk away, their dreams mangled. Auditions are cruel.

Before travelling to TCD that morning, I was confident that I could perform my monologues well. I thought I had a reasonable chance of getting through the actual acting part of the audition. It was the 'movement' session that I was worried about. When I was just doing random drama exercises, I never felt in control like I did when I was onstage. My experiences at the Young Gaiety had taught me that I wasn't very good at the type of 'movement' that drama instructors usually wanted you to engage in. This was partly because I felt so self-conscious while doing the 'movement'. What went on later that afternoon in Trinity could have been plucked right out of *Monty Python*.

Shortly after half past two, the seven other remaining applicants and I were taken back to the blue-floored rehearsal area. We were asked to remove our footwear. I took off my shoes, foot brace, and socks.

There were three instructors in the room — two men and Chrissie. It was one of the men — a slim, light-footed fellow — who took charge of the session. The other instructors merely sat behind a desk and observed, silently judging us.

First, the man in charge told us to jog around the room in various ways — normally, sideways, backwards . . . Soon, however, he stopped telling us to jog. 'Now, just find your own space,' he invited.

Then came the really surreal part.

'Okay,' the instructor began, 'I want you to imagine you've got a tennis ball in your pelvis. That's right. Now, just rotate the tennis ball gently around your pelvis . . .'

I started moving my hips in circles.

'Okay, now the tennis ball is speeding up . . .'

I moved my hips faster.

'Now it's slowing down again.'

I eased back to a calmer pace.

'Right, now the tennis ball is moving up your abdomen, up into your chest, into your neck, into your head . . . That's right. Now just rotate it gently around your head . . . That's it . . . Okay, now it's going into your left arm, down to your wrist, rotate it around your wrist . . . Very good . . . Now it's moving to your right shoulder, down your right arm . . .'

As I twisted my body to his instructions, I couldn't help thinking I would have been better equipped to cope had I smoked something rather potent before the session.

'Okay, now the tennis ball is rolling down into your right leg, down into your foot, twirl it around your ankle.'

The pain almost made me stop.

'Now the tennis ball is boiling hot.'

I pretended my internal organs were burning.

'Now the tennis ball is icy cold.'

I acted as if my insides were freezing.

'Now there are two tennis balls.'

I couldn't keep up!

Eventually, the tennis balls were expelled through our fingertips. And the session was over.

The seven other course-applicants and I put our footwear back on. Then we went into an adjoining room, and waited.

The minutes went by. Finally, Chrissie arrived. She pointed to the three people she and her fellow instructors had selected to go on to the next round.

I was not one of them.

I wandered out of the building in a daze. A BAS student who was sitting by the door said to me as I made my way passed her, 'You can try again next year!'

I tried to smile.

Of course, even those who continued to Round Three that afternoon were not guaranteed a Bachelor in Acting Studies place. They went on to a one-on-one session with an instructor. In a few weeks, they would each receive a letter that would either offer them a place, invite them to a further audition, or inform them that they hadn't been accepted this year.

But I would receive no such letter of any kind. My quest had ended.

I felt rejected, worthless. I trudged through the Trinity campus, and sat down on a wooden bench by the edge of College Park. A tree above was covering me in its shade. There were clumps of people dotted around the perimeter of the sharply green grass. It was a sickeningly sunny afternoon.

I took a box of cigarettes and a lighter from my coat pocket, put one of the white sticks into my mouth, and lit it. Since smoking my first cigarette over a year before, I hadn't become a heavy smoker. I still didn't really think of myself as a 'smoker' at all. I smoked about two cigarettes a month, and I usually only lit up when I was with friends who also smoked. I don't know why I kept up the habit. I knew that smoking while having Fanconi anaemia was a complete no-no. I guess it was a comfort, sometimes. I felt safer knowing that comfort was available on days like this.

The night after my BAS audition, I rang Gerard to tell him I'd failed to get a place. My uncle lifted my spirits a little by saying that he thought getting through the actual acting round was quite good for a first-timer. Gerard advised me to audition for a BAS place again the following summer, and to spend the time up until then 'reading plays and partying'.

But I didn't fancy putting my life on hold for twelve months, simply to gamble for a BAS place again. I felt directionless. I still had a shot at getting a Drama and Theatre Studies place, of course, but I wasn't sure I wanted one anymore. I didn't feel like heading straight into a third-level academic course — not just after the Leaving Cert. I was fed up of study, of exams.

I talked about these things with Gina MacDonnell, when I finally got to see her. Two days after my BAS audition, I paid her a visit in Our Lady's.

I talked about many other things with Gina that afternoon, as well; what a relief it was to be over the Leaving Cert; how brilliant it had been to win Best Actor at the One-Act; the perpetual loneliness and sadness which plagued me.

'Sadness is my default emotion,' I told Gina, smiling.

The psychologist nodded slowly. 'I feel like I kind of abandoned you after the transplant,' she said. 'We haven't met since then.'

'I never felt abandoned,' I said. 'After the transplant, I needed time to myself.'

'And now?' Gina asked.

I was silent. I knew what I wanted to say, but saying each word was still like pushing a jumbo jet uphill.

'I think a big part of the reason I'm so lonely,' I began, 'is that for six years I have been in love with someone who has never loved me back.'

There was a pause.

'Emma,' Gina said.

I remembered the collection of writings I had put together in May 2002 — the collection dedicated to Emma. I'd posted a copy to Gina. I suppose it wouldn't have been too difficult for a psychologist to glean my true feelings from the pieces therein.

'Yes,' I replied.

'Why is the love unrequited?' Gina asked. 'Is it because Emma doesn't know? Or . . .'

'She knows,' I said. 'She just doesn't feel the same way. And, of course, I accept that. It's just . . .' I closed my eyes to hold in the tears, but one ambled down my cheek regardless. 'I've gone through so much pain because of her.'

Silence, again.

'We all, at some point in our lives,' Gina began, 'reach a time when we need to talk to someone, someone outside our immediate environment. I think maybe you're at that stage of your life right now.'

I nodded. 'Can you help me?' I said.

17. A friend, a holiday, and some results

A few days after my BAS audition, I met up with Aisling in Bray.

After I left St Andrew's, I had sent her an email, expressing my hope that our friendship could continue into the future. Since the *Teechers* cast party, Aisling and I had grown close quickly. In fact, her friendship was becoming invaluable to me.

On that July afternoon, the pair of us meandered around Bray for a while, simply sharing our thoughts. After this, I travelled with Aisling and her parents into the Wicklow wilderness. We went to the property of some friends of theirs, to pick blackcurrants.

I told Aisling that I'd failed to get a Bachelor in Acting Studies place.

'Well, it's their loss,' she said.

Aisling always said the right thing. She had a way of making me feel better by just being there.

As Aisling and I sat in a tree's shadow that July evening, sunlight pouring over everything except us, she described in glowing terms her recent holiday in Cuba.

After she'd exhausted this topic, she told me that it was my turn to ramble on for a while. I couldn't think of anything to ramble on about, however. So Aisling asked me to tell her the story of my bone marrow transplant.

I related the tale as best I could.

When I'd finished, Aisling looked at me.

'You meet these people,' she began, 'and before you even know too much about them, you know there's something inspirational about them. You are one of those incredible people, Ben.'

I laughed, embarrassed.

'Well, thank you, Aisling,' I managed. 'You're pretty incredible too.'

On 14 July 2003, I set off for New York City. Mai, Bing, and I were going on a two-week holiday. This was to be my third visit to America, but my first to the Big Apple.

On the morning of the 14th, we departed from Dublin Airport. Our flight was delayed, however, as we had to wait on the runway while the bags of a passenger who had never boarded were removed from the cargo hold. Concern over terrorism was obviously high. And we were going to the city where terrorists had jolted those fears to the forefront of everyone's mind.

One of the first things I noticed about New York was how raw the emotional wounds of 9/11 still were. As we travelled in a taxi from JFK International Airport to our rented apartment in Manhattan's West Village, our driver spoke openly about his experiences that day.

My mum, on the other hand, nattered about how she had lived and worked in New York some thirty years earlier, while the World Trade Center towers were being built.

'Wow,' the cabdriver exclaimed, 'that's, like, before I was born!'

The apartment Mai, Bing, and I stayed in in the West Village could have been considered either cosy or cluttered, depending on your viewpoint. It was the home of an artist/photographer, who was living out of town for a while. The walls were covered with her own photography and painting, and most of the floor was hidden under three-foot-high stacks of thick, hardback books.

Apparently, this woman's subletting her apartment was a little bit illegal. Mum talked to her before we left for the States and, during that phone call, the artist/photographer asked that, while we were staying in the apartment, Mai, Bing, and I pretend we were relations of hers from Europe.

The apartment came with a computer, and broadband Internet access. Aisling and I wrote long emails to each other during the two weeks I was in NYC. It was wonderful to come back to the apartment after a day of seeing grand sights, and read the random thoughts of a close friend. When I returned from New York, the long emails continued throughout the summer holidays, even though Aisling and I lived only a few miles apart.

Mai, Bing, and I saw a lot of what NY had to offer during our visit—the museums, the Empire State Building, Ellis Island, Liberty Island, Chinatown, Little Italy, and, of course, Ground Zero. As we approached the 'hole in the ground', as some of the locals called it, we passed street vendors selling 9/11 photo albums, t-shirts, and other souvenirs. It was a terrifically warm day, but the whole area around where the towers had been was chilling. I couldn't help feeling like a voyeur as I peered through the metal fencing at the mass grave that was now a construction site.

Sightseeing and soaking up culture were all very well. But the most interesting experience of our New York holiday happened in our rented apartment. Well, right outside our rented apartment. The three of us arrived back one evening to find an eviction notice taped to the door.

The notice was, thankfully, not intended for us, but for the owner. She was allegedly a few payments behind in her rent.

All told, my fortnight in New York was a great escape from the mundanity of Kilmacanogue.

On a clear Wednesday morning in mid-August 2003, I travelled to St Andrew's College by DART with a bunch of friends.

It was Leaving Cert results day.

When we arrived at Andrew's, we all went to the school's reception desk, where we were each handed a sealed brown envelope. I walked back out to the air, and then tore open my envelope.

I pulled out the slip of paper that was inside, searching for that all-important points number.

I'd got 510 points.

But there were no A1s.

I had to console myself by insisting that I couldn't have done any more work and at the same time stayed sane.

Besides, it wasn't as if these results were bad.

My Andrew's friends and I went to a movie after we'd got our results. After the movie, we went for a meal, and then indulged in the obligatory night of drunkenness.

The following week, the CAO Round One college offers came out.

I was offered a Drama and Theatre Studies place. The final points requirement for the course was exactly 510.

But I wasn't going to be accepting the place I'd been offered. At least, not this year. I wrote to Trinity College, pleading for a deferral. A year's deferral would allow me to take up my place in October

2004, without having to go through the points lottery all over again. In my letter to TCD, I explained that I'd had a bone marrow transplant two years before, and that this had led to my spending a year out of school. I wrote that I needed time to 'prepare for the new challenges' I would face at university. It was all very serious stuff.

Trinity didn't have to grant me a deferral. But they did.

So I was now on a 'gap year', a 'year out'. I was finished with second-level education, and I wouldn't be beginning third level for at least fourteen months or so. Over a year of empty days was stretching out before me.

What the hell was I going to do with myself?

18. Maybe not forever

On a Wednesday afternoon in August '03, my therapy sessions with Gina began.

Gina's office in the psychology wing of Our Lady's Hospital for Sick Children was a strange setting for the quite adult discussions we would end up having. There was no therapist's couch. I sat in a swivel chair by Gina's desk; she sat in the corner opposite me, her back to a window. There were cartoon-character stickers stuck to the walls, and children's toys were piled up on a low table to my right.

My parents didn't ask too many questions when I told them that Gina thought I needed some therapy. Mai and Des figured it was about time I talked to someone about my transplant, and about the other things I'd experienced because of Fanconi anaemia. I don't think they suspected that my illness was not going to be the focus of the sessions.

'I feel like Tony Soprano,' I said on my first day, as I nestled myself into the chair opposite Gina.

That joke didn't sum up my real feelings. I felt guilty about being in therapy. I felt weak, unable to deal with my own sorrows.

The first thing she and I talked about was Emma. And, once I started talking, I actually found it hard to halt the flow. Over the next few sessions, Gina would frequently accuse me of 'intellectualising' my emotions. But, as far as I was concerned, talking about emotions at all meant intellectualising them. I didn't know any other way to explain myself.

'I did all those things lovesick people do,' I told Gina on that first Wednesday afternoon. 'I dialled her number and then hung up the phone before she answered. I read her letters over and over. I kissed the place where she'd signed her name on the letters. I heard her in every love song.

'But Emma and I can joke about stuff like that now,' I continued. 'You know, I might say, "Remember that time I was stalking you", or something.'

I laughed.

'Is Emma a very good-looking girl?' Gina asked.

'Yes.'

'Do you think your feelings were mainly a physical thing?'

'No,' I answered, perhaps a little too quickly. 'Well, I mean, I never let myself think about her in a crude way.'

'Was that not a bit naïve?' Gina pressed. 'I mean, what did you want from this girl if you didn't want a romantic, a potentially sexual, relationship?'

'Well, don't get me wrong,' I responded, 'I mean, I'm a teenage guy, and I have the same kind of urges as every other teenage guy, but . . . Well, first of all, Emma was more important to me than that. And then, honestly, I didn't really think about sex that much. I thought it'd be nice to have it and stuff — but I always had my trusty left hand,' I laughed, holding that hand up.

'I didn't think about a sexual relationship with Emma,' I said. 'I thought about a physical relationship with her — holding her hand, having her arms around me. That's what I thought about, that's what I dreamt about. Someone I loved to hold me through everything.'

I went on, 'I think, on reflection, my illness had a lot to do with the intensity of my feelings for Emma. I mean, having Fanconi anaemia made me feel isolated and alone to start with, and then I suppose I was clinging to the only romantic experience I'd ever had.

'And it was when I was coming up to my transplant that I just had to tell her that I loved her, because I was afraid that if I didn't . . . well, I mightn't get another chance.'

I told Gina that that moment on the phone in March 2001 was probably the only truly spontaneous moment of my life.

I then described the worst aspect of loving Emma unrequitedly. 'I couldn't stop thinking about her,' I said. 'It was as if I were constantly drowning in my feelings for her.

'But it wasn't just because I was in love with her that I couldn't stop thinking about her. It's the way my mind works. I don't know how other people think, but I obsess, I over-analyse. I find it so hard to stop thinking about things.'

Gina later described the way I thought as being like obsessive-compulsive disorder, without the compulsive part. In other words, I obsessed over stuff in my own head, but this rarely affected my outward behaviour.

'I suppose,' I continued, 'I do feel more disconnected from my love for Emma now than I ever have. It's still there—I still love her with everything inside me. But I don't want to have these feelings anymore; I don't want to cling to them anymore. I'm trying to find a way to get rid of them.

'Even coming out of love is hard, though. It's become so much a part of who I thought I was. Without it, I almost don't know who I am.

'And I still feel so lonely.'

I glanced at the floor. 'When I think of all the days and nights that I spent just sitting, desperately wanting to be with Emma yet knowing I couldn't. When you want something that badly, you feel you almost have it.'

On 1 September 2003, I went to my aunt and uncle's house in Killiney, Co. Dublin. I would be staying there for two weeks. My aunt and uncle were paying me to housesit, while they holidayed in France.

It was a pretty terrific situation, really—I had a house all to myself, and I was getting money for being there! This was my first proper taste of independent living—I had to shop for myself, cook for myself, leave out the rubbish bags . . .

This taste of independence also coincided with something else that made me feel very grown up. Hair had been growing on my chin, cheeks, and upper lip for several months. But, one morning during those two weeks in Killiney, the sight of the light brown fuzz became too much to bear. I bought a razor and shaving foam, and had my first shave. I guess I was pretty late to develop the beginnings of a beard, compared to my peers. I was by this time nearly nineteen, after all. Fanconi anaemia will slow you down like that, though.

A lot of my time in Killiney, I spent writing. I was doing the usual stuff—*Totally Fushed*, poetry. This kind of writing had been a welcome distraction during my school days, and I still enjoyed it. But, now that I had more free time than ever before, I was also searching for a bigger project.

'Why don't you write your story?' proposed John Douglas, my one-time English tutor, one afternoon. 'I think that'd be a good thing to do.'

'How was your week?'

This was the question with which Gina began every therapy session, as I continued to visit her throughout September.

'Fine' was my usual reply. Or, 'Good.' Or, once, 'I'm excited about the upcoming Democratic primaries in the US. I'm hoping they'll pick someone who can get rid of Bush.'

One afternoon, Gina asked me, 'What's it like to be Ben? Because I've been reading over some of the writing you gave me, and sometimes I'll read something and say to myself, "I wish I could write like that", but then I think that to write the things you do, you'd have to have gone through a lot of pain.'

I smiled. 'It's good to be Ben,' I said. 'Sometimes there has been pain,' I accepted. 'But hopefully that makes you a better writer, or a better actor, better able to affect people. I always want to be affecting people, even if it's just my own friends. That's why I'm always working on some project, be it an issue of the magazine, or whatever.

'I think there are two kinds of happiness,' I told Gina. 'Achievement-based happiness, and personal happiness — happiness in your personal life. I've always seen the former as being far more important than the latter.'

According to my worldview, the goal of one's life was not to be happy, but to achieve one's potential at whatever cost to personal happiness.

'It's just that,' I continued, 'sometimes, it's hard to go on without being personally happy!'

My psychologist asked why I wasn't working as hard on my personal happiness as I was on my achievement-based happiness.

'I don't know how to do that,' I conceded.

Gina seemed to think that, now that I was healthy and had my body back to myself, I should be embracing life's carnal pleasures. But that had never been me.

'I don't really like nightclubs, or those kinds of things,' I said. 'I mean, I can tolerate them if I have to. But I get nervous around groups of people. I even get scared going into shops!'

'How can you on the one hand love the stage and love the attention that you get from being onstage, and on the other hand be scared of walking into a shop?' Gina asked.

'It's about control,' I explained. 'When I'm onstage I know who

I'm supposed to be. When I'm just out in public, nobody's given me a role and that makes me frightened of how people will judge me.

'See, while I've always had a massive ego, I don't think I've ever had much self-confidence.

'I mean, there's a part of me that . . . ' I smiled. 'Well, if all the kings, queens, presidents, and prime ministers on the planet came to me tomorrow and said "Ben, we've decided to make you King of the World", this part of me would wonder why they weren't making me King of the Universe!' I laughed. 'But then, there's a part of me that's just terrified of simple things like walking down the street.'

While I may have been nervous around groups of people, when I was with just one person, I was fine, I told Gina. When I was with just one person, I could 'scan' what that person wanted from me, and put up an act to suit his or her personality.

'I don't know how to be natural,' I said to my psychologist. 'I only know how to act natural.'

Gina described me as a 'social chameleon', but I resented this label.

'I don't see it as being disingenuous,' I protested. 'I'm just trying to make people happy.'

I told my therapist that putting on these slightly different personas had enabled me to form close friendships with many different kinds of people.

'I even talk differently depending on the friends I'm with,' I admitted, 'I use different vocabularies.'

'How can you say you're not a social chameleon?!' Gina exclaimed.

'Well, I don't know, maybe I am,' I conceded. 'But I'm not trying to be someone I'm not. I'm all the Bens.'

Gina suggested that, as long as I was trying to be what I thought others wanted me to be, I would never find the personal happiness I pined for.

'How can you have any real closeness in your life?' she asked.

'But I do have closeness!' I insisted. 'With so many different kinds of friends. I've just never found the person who can fight away all my sadness and loneliness. Maybe I'm asking for too much. But then, I thought for so long that I knew who that person was. I knew I couldn't have her, but I still saw her as the answer to all that I didn't like about my life.' I smiled. 'How do you let go of a goddess?'

In the last week of September, I began working at my dad's account-ancy practice in Monkstown, Co. Dublin.

Des and his business partner set up this practice in 1979. The first 'office' they occupied was merely a room in a house in Donnybrook, Dublin. They had two desks and a couple of chairs between them, and they had to use the payphone in the hall to contact clients. Des had left one of the top accountancy firms of the day, where he was an Assistant Manager, because he wanted to work with small and me-dium-sized businesses rather than big companies.

From those beginnings in Donnybrook, Des and his partner's firm grew into a fairly successful operation. The firm moved location a few times, before settling in Monkstown in 1998.

What Des wanted me to do for him in the autumn of '03 was cre-ate a new filing system for his office. The old one was banjaxed, thanks to years of files being put back in the wrong places. Thankfully, I had prior experience with filing. During the summer of 2000, I did a cou-ple of days' work in UCD for our neighbour, the lecturer. I spent those days sorting research papers—and getting introduced to peo-ple, such as the wispy-haired professor walking around with his fly unzipped.

In Des's office, I spent my first day and a half shredding docu-ments. I then moved outside to the 'sheds'. These concrete, bunker-like buildings were filled with thousands of files. It was here, amidst the dried leaves, the cobwebs, the cigarette butts, and the rat poison, that the real file-sorting began. I worked from 9 a.m. to 5.30 p.m. on Mondays, Tuesdays, Thursdays, and Fridays. On Wednesdays, I only worked till lunchtime. Then I went off to see Gina.

I wouldn't say my job was 'fun', exactly. On particularly cold days, I used to look in at the other employees through one of the outside windows, and wonder what it would be like to have a desk job. Still, I couldn't complain—my dad was saving me from having to go out and actually look for employment. And, at the very least, working in Des's office came with fringe benefits. It allowed me to take the DART every morning with Aisling, who was now in Sixth Year in St Andrew's.

I remember the chilly September morning I first took the train with Aisling. As we stepped onto the carriage, she presented me with a huge bar of chocolate, and a jar of jam. She'd bought the chocolate during a recent trip to England, and the jam was made from the black-currants we picked in July.

One lunchtime shortly after I began my job as my dad's 'Archive Technician', I was sitting with Des in an Italian restaurant near his office. He was eating a pizza; I was gobbling spaghetti Bolognese, consuming the dish, as I usually did, systematically — eating the meat off the top first, then eating the pasta underneath.

Des told me that I was coming into work too early. I was arriving in Monkstown at about 8.30 each morning, but the employee who kept the keys to the sheds didn't arrive at the office till nine o'clock. Every morning, I was spending half an hour just sitting around.

'Why don't you walk Aisling up to school before coming to the office?' Des suggested. 'That's what I'd do if I were in your position.'

That evening, I asked Aisling whether she would mind my walking up to Andrew's with her. She assured me that she would 'really enjoy' my company.

So, from that point on, I walked up to school with Aisling each weekday morning.

The pair of us talked about everything on those walks. Sometimes, we even talked about nothing. Silences were just another part of the conversation.

We seemed to laugh a lot, as well.

I quickly became attached to this routine. I'd never felt so at ease around another person. Aisling was teaching me that I didn't have to be anybody but Ben, whoever Ben was on any given day.

As these mornings went on, I realised what this girl had become to me: my best friend.

One cold autumn morning, as we passed through the St Andrew's main gate, I developed a furious urge to tell Aisling all these things. But it was not the time.

Instead, I simply said, 'I want to thank you.'

Aisling laughed. 'For what?'

I put my hand on her arm. 'You're a big part of the reason why I'm happier now than I was . . . even up to a few months ago.'

She smiled. 'I've learnt so much from you as well,' she said. 'And I'm glad that you're happy now.'

I grinned. 'Happier,' I jokingly corrected.

Aisling laughed again. 'Well,' she said, 'I don't think any of us are ever . . .' she grinned comically, and swayed her arms in a kind of happy dance.

I smiled. 'No,' I agreed.

We exchanged goodbyes, and she went into school.

I left the Andrew's grounds through the rear gate, and then went back down to Booterstown DART Station, to catch a train to Monkstown.

Such was my routine during these, the best mornings of my life.

As October began, I started talking to Gina about Aisling, and how her friendship had affected me.

'All the things admirable about humanity, you will find in Aisling,' I told my therapist. 'Compassion, drive, talent,' I went on.

'That's high praise,' said Gina.

It was. But Aisling deserved it.

At an evening concert in St Andrew's around this time, Aisling played a flute solo, and accompanied on piano the school choir.

I remember, on the morning before the concert, while Aisling and I were on the DART together, I was humming the Beatles' 'Yesterday' to myself. I thought I heard a whimper of recognition from Aisling, but she didn't say anything. 'Yesterday' then turned out to be one of the songs she played at the concert.

I never went to a school concert during my time as a St Andrew's student. So it was nice to go back and experience this aspect of the school's extracurricular life—even as an observer. As a kid, I had a brief dalliance with the violin. But I gave it up once I realised that I was never going to be very good. Music was something I didn't understand, something otherworldly, a kind of magic. The people who could understand and use music's power were magicians.

After the concert, I stood near the St Andrew's reception area, waiting for Aisling to leave the main hall. When she emerged through the blue doors, I went up to her.

'Can I have your autograph?' I asked, grinning.

She smiled. 'Oh, I don't know about that, now.'

As Aisling and I chatted, a man I hadn't seen in some time approached us.

'Ah,' Mr Agnew began, surveying Aisling and me, 'my two students who never wear!'

Mr Agnew congratulated Aisling on her powerful playing, and invited her to perform at a concert he was organising for the following spring. The purpose of this concert was to impress envoys from American universities who would be visiting St Andrew's.

Aisling tentatively accepted Mr A's invitation, and then went off to talk to her mum.

'So, are you in college now?' Mr Agnew asked me.

'No,' I said. I told him that I'd deferred taking up the Drama and Theatre place I'd been offered.

Mr Agnew seemed to approve of my decision. 'It's good to be a bit older when you go to college,' he said.

'Yeah,' I agreed. 'At the moment, I'm just working with my dad, but I'd like to do some serious writing this year.'

Mr Agnew grinned. 'Or some serious editing.'

I smiled. 'What was it you always told us, sir? "The essence of writing is rewriting"?'

He laughed. 'Well, it's true,' he said. 'It's true.'

'I don't know,' I mused, 'if I ever do go into writing as a career, I'll probably be doing political pieces or something.'

'The next Fintan O'Toole,' Mr Agnew joked. Mr A then told me that he'd read something about one of Mr O'Toole's former teachers. Apparently the teacher had not remembered Fintan being in his class.

'But I will always remember you, Ben,' Mr Agnew said, in his inimitably droll tone.

'Well, thank you, sir.'

Over the next few months, I contributed articles to a couple of websites, and I penned what I considered to be my first 'proper' poetry. My earlier poems had waffled a lot; now I wanted to capture a moment, or an emotion, as concisely and accurately as possible. Poetry is the space between feeling and knowing. Those words on the page have to reveal some corner of your heart—to you, and hopefully to others too. I felt that I was now, at last, beginning to make some headway.

Toward the end of 2003, I received a letter commenting on some of my work from Thomas Kinsella. Mr Kinsella's daughter had visited our house during the summer. She was friendly with my mum, as they were doing the same course in UCD. Mr Kinsella's daughter suggested I give her some poems to pass on to her father. She warned me, however, that he would not sugarcoat his words: 'You'll get the truth.'

In his letter, Thomas Kinsella offered much-needed constructive criticism. But he also told me that some of my work constituted 'a very good start', and he advised me to 'certainly' keep writing verse, to keep 'excavating those important memories, feelings and opinions'. Finally, Mr Kinsella wished me luck 'on the hard road'. It was a privilege to get such a letter.

I soon got a taste of the 'hard road' that Thomas Kinsella had mentioned. A few months after I received TK's letter, the first poems I sent to a poetry magazine were rejected. 'There are some good things here,' the editors of the magazine wrote on the rejection slip, 'but these are not quite right for our publication.'

Of course, rejection is part of every writer's growing pains. John Douglas urged me to take it all in my stride.

'Don't write for them,' he advised. 'Write for yourself.'

His remark reminded me of something I'd read in one of Rainer Maria Rilke's *Letters to a Young Poet*. Rilke asks writers to ask themselves whether they must write.

I must write. Were I forced to renounce writing, I would without doubt have to die.

I learned much about the craft of writing during my year out. I learned things through trial and error in my own work; I also got to interview poet Eamon Grennan and writer/broadcaster Bill Long for *Totally Fushed*, and I learned from both of them. Mr Long told me that the biggest sin with regard to writing was to 'rush things'. 'Hurry,' he said, 'spoils a lot of artists. Hurry, and you could put in brackets after that: money. And I think hurry comes from wanting money.'

Years before our interview, Bill Long was the recipient of a heart transplant. He had a camera crew follow him through the procedure, and the footage was edited to create a documentary for RTÉ called *A Change of Heart*. He also wrote a book of the same name.

Bill and I laughed as we compared 'pill counts'. 'Looking back on it,' Bill said of his transplant experience, 'not so much now, but looking back on it two or three years after, I used to say to myself, "How did I manage to do that?" But it's extraordinary, when you're in the situation, it's very different. It's like looking at somebody else's transplant.'

The next time I saw Aisling play in an organised setting was at the St Andrew's College Prize Giving in November 2003. This was held at Jurys Hotel in Ballsbridge.

The atmosphere of Prize Night was always oppressively formal. The whole thing was a bit like a religious ceremony. The night would begin with a procession of fully robed teachers, moving sombrely as monks, for which we'd all have to stand. Then various St Andrew's dignitaries would rise to engage in a little self-love, lauding the school and its achievements. The audience would always politely titter at the jokes in the speeches, like churchgoers who knew when to say 'Amen'.

On Prize Night 2003, I was given an award for English, and one for German, because I'd got Leaving Cert Higher Level A2s in both subjects. It was a pleasant enough evening. I got a chance to chat with classmates I thought I'd never see again. And, of course, I got to watch Aisling play during one of the musical interludes. There was even a certain nostalgic feel about the oppressive formality. This was the last time I'd see this tradition in action.

Besides, no matter what the context, it's always nice when someone gives you an award. Gratifying as they were to receive, however, the academic accolades St Andrew's presented me with could not compare with what I considered to be the greatest triumph of my life.

It happened during Sixth Class. Every year, BSP—like a lot of schools—held a Sports Day. Now, I'd never been good at sports, and, of course, I wasn't allowed to play contact sports. But, as Sixth Class began, I was becoming quite a fast runner. One of the fastest in my class, in fact.

In the summer term of '97, I got through the pre-Sports Day sprint heats for my age group (over-elevens or under-thirteens, I can't recall) for the first time. And then, on Sports Day itself, I joined the other sprint finalists at the starting line of the grass 'track' in the Bray field where every BSP Sports Day was held.

My dad says he remembers me loosening my muscles before the race by shaking my legs, like I'd seen athletes do on TV. Des was a big athletics fan, and sometimes the two of us watched the sport together.

One of the BSP teachers yelled 'Ready . . . Set . . . Go!' And I sped off. I pushed my legs as hard as I could; my breath came in short gasps, the finish line was all I could see.

I won the bronze medal in that race. When I was presented with my award, I raised my fist to greet the cheers. Coming third in the BSP under-thirteens (or over-elevens) sprint was the proudest moment of my life at that point. And I still cherish my medal today, though my head no longer fits through the ribbon.

Of course, I was on anabolic steroids at the time. So, if it had been the Olympics, I would have been disqualified. But I don't like to talk about that part.

Getting therapy in Gina's child-orientated office was an odd experience. But it was also odd visiting Crumlin Hospital every week for a reason other than to be poked with needles.

In the summer of 2003, I had my second annual post-BMT battery of tests. Having had my first post-BMT battery a year before, I knew what to expect. The post-BMT batteries were a lot like the pre-BMT battery — they involved the scanning and prodding of various parts of my body.

The 2003 tests confirmed that, physically, I was doing better than ever. But I wasn't entirely out of the woods. Chronic GVHD has been known to appear in patients up to three years after a transplant. There were also, of course, ongoing concerns that I might develop some form of cancer. Not long after the battery, I received an email from someone at the Fanconi Anemia Research Fund, reminding me of 'the risk of squamous cell carcinoma in FA patients'. The risk of an FA patient developing this form of cancer increases as the patient gets older. In terms of the non-bone-marrow-related worries of Fanconi anaemia, I would never be out of the woods.

But, while I was well, I could believe that I would be well forever. There didn't seem to be any other way to live. I wasn't about to let worry waste my days.

After my '03 battery, my regular checkups in Our Lady's were reduced to twice a year.

It was strange going back to St John's, sometimes — seeing the medical staff I used to see much more often. Maybe it was just the way I felt about myself, but I felt like the doctors and nurses expected something from me. I was one of their success stories. They expected me to succeed in the new life I'd been given.

I'd been going to John's for ten years, over half my life. I'd grown up while attending that ward. I'd seen staff join and leave; I'd known doctors from all over the world. I almost felt like I owned the ward. Strange though it was, it was also a comfort to return to John's.

By this time, however, I was well past the age at which I should have stopped attending a children's hospital. Aengus constantly spoke of transferring me to St James's, but kept making excuses not to do it.

'You have a relationship with Gina, which I don't want to jeopardise,' he told me on one occasion.

Eventually, Aengus settled on saying that I could come to Crumlin for my infrequent checkups for the foreseeable future. If I ever fell ill again, though, I would need to be admitted to James's. He joked that my Crumlin trips would be 'social calls', 'probably more for my benefit than yours!'

'I'll bring beer,' I laughed.

'But I'm always here if you need me,' he went on. 'Or if you want to give me presents or anything.'

One afternoon, Aengus and I were sitting in that old consultancy room in St John's, and he asked me what my plans were regarding college, etc. I told him the story with my Drama and Theatre place; then I mentioned my Bachelor in Acting Studies audition, and told him that I'd performed monologues from *Macbeth* and *The Norman Conquests*.

Aengus told me that his brother-in-law was an actor, and that he'd once gone to see him in a production of *Macbeth*.

'But I couldn't tell what was going on,' Dr O'Marcaigh admitted. 'Someone got stabbed or something. Anyway, I went to the pub across the road and read the *Evening Herald* and had a much better time.'

Just think — this man saves children's lives while under great strain every day, but ask him to sit through one of the greatest plays in the English language . . . 'I find unrelated bone marrow transplantation easier than Shakespeare any day,' he concluded.

I left Crumlin that afternoon feeling like I knew Aengus just that little bit better. My twice-yearly visits really were getting like social calls.

Thankfully, then, I had other hospitals to go to, where proper 'health' business was conducted. Our Lady's wasn't the only place I still visited for checkups. Every year since the removal of the growth on my tongue, I've had to return to the Dental Hospital to see Dr Flint.

During one visit to the Dental Hospital, I was finally given a reason for the perpetual dryness of my mouth. Since the start of the problem in 2002, I hadn't really thought of telling Dr Flint about it. It didn't even occur to me that Dr Flint was a mouth doctor—this was his area of expertise.

But then, during this particular checkup at the Dental Hospital, I was asked whether I was having any problems with my mouth, and I mentioned the constant thirst. Dr Flint conducted a little test. He gave me a white beaker, and told me to spit into it every few seconds for five minutes. Then he and his scrubs-wearing posse swished out of the room, and I was left sitting alone in the dentist's chair, holding and spitting into my white cup.

Soon, Dr Flint and his gang of straight-faced students returned. He had brought another consultant with him, as well.

'This is Ben,' my doctor said to the other consultant, 'the boy I butchered!' Dr Flint flashed me a grin. He told me the other doctor's name, and the other doctor shook my hand.

Dr Flint continued, 'Ben's case was very unusual, because . . .' He went on to detail my medical history to the other consultant, before giving his reasons for removing the white growth from my tongue. 'As I say, because of an imminent bone marrow transplant.'

The other consultant nodded, concurring with Dr Flint that getting rid of the growth had been the prudent course of action.

'We were in uncharted waters with Ben here.' Dr Flint smiled again. 'And that's why Ben's in our atlas! Have you seen our atlas, Ben?'

'No,' I said.

Dr Flint produced a thick, hardback book, and flicked through the pages until he found a particular one. 'There you are,' he said, handing me the tome and pointing to a pair of photographs.

While the patient's name did not appear beneath the photos, the pictures showed my tongue, before and after the procedure Dr Flint had performed on it.

It was nice to discover that, even when I was not physically present at the Dental Hospital, I could still be used as a learning tool.

After the spit in my beaker had been measured, Dr Flint suggested that my salivary glands were producing a less-than-average amount of saliva. He speculated that this was probably because my glands had been damaged by my pre-BMT total body irradiation.

Dr Flint said that there was a drug I could take to try and combat my dry mouth, and he wrote me a prescription. He warned, however, that the side effects of this drug included constant sweating and persistent diarrhoea.

'You really just have to experiment with the dosage,' he said, 'until you find a balance between the side effects and the dryness in your mouth.'

Given that the dryness in my mouth wasn't debilitating, just annoying, the whole 'see how much sweating and diarrhoea you can tolerate' experiment was not something I was too willing to try. Dr Flint's prescription from that day remains, unfilled, on my desk in my room.

Clearly, visiting the Dental Hospital was a bit strange at times — but I liked seeing Dr Flint once a year. It was nice to be able to keep contact with doctors who had helped me.

On one of my six-monthly checkups in Crumlin, I bumped into another doctor who had helped me — Dr Neil Adamson. 'How are you?' he asked.

On many afternoons throughout the final month of my BMT, Dr Adamson had sat with me in my room. He would ask me questions about my life and I'd try to answer. Gina and Dr Adamson had my back during that time.

'I'm well.'

'Are you still keeping up your magazine and your writing?'

I told him I was. I then asked how he was doing.

He said he was busy. He was trying to organise more government funding for Our Lady's.

This reminded me of something another Crumlin consultant had once told me. He said he found it amusing that he and other Our Lady's staff could lobby ministers for ages, stressing how dire the situation in the hospital was, but it wasn't until patients and their parents started telling their horror stories to the press that additional funds actually started coming in.

I always thought that was a revealing comment. Not so much with regard to the motives of politicians, but with regard to the power of patients and parents to really make a difference. While I knew and had seen the horrors of the Irish health service, I personally couldn't claim to be a victim of government under-funding. Indeed, government funds are the reason I'm alive today. The approximate total cost of my bone marrow transplant was €200,000, and the vast majority of that bill was paid by the taxpayers.

The issue of funding, though, and of how best to persuade the government to give more money, was always an important one at Our Lady's. I remember one day back in 2000, sitting in the St John's waiting area, having a blood transfusion. The then Minister for Health, Micheál Martin, was due to visit Our Lady's that afternoon, and there had been some debate among the consultants and administrative staff over whether beds should be removed from the hallways. If they were removed, the hospital would look more presentable; if they were left in the hallways, a more accurate impression of the state of affairs in Our Lady's would be given. In the end, I think they moved the beds.

When Minister Martin arrived at St John's, Dr Breathnach, who was guiding him around, introduced him to my dad and me. I stood up and shook his hand.

'Minister,' I said. In spite of myself, I felt my nerves in my knees. This was a powerful man — a man I'd seen on TV.

The Minister for Health offered a look of concern. And then he and his dark-suited aides continued on their whirlwind tour.

Throughout my hours of therapy with Dr Gina MacDonnell, we didn't discuss my illness much. What could I say? It was there, stuck to me like a part of myself. Growing up for me was growing up with Fanconi anaemia. My illness had brought pain, of course, but I was also sure that it had influenced me in myriad undetectable ways.

'I guess I became almost protective of this illness in the run-up to my transplant,' I told Gina one day. 'Protective of myself with this illness. If people slagged me or laughed at me, I felt I was being persecuted because I had FA.'

Gina asked if I was angry about having Fanconi anaemia.

'No,' I said. It wasn't an entirely truthful response. Of course there were times when anger crept into my thoughts, when I felt bitter about having this life-threatening disease, and about everything my mind and body had been dragged through because of it. But I tried not to project this image to the world. And I hated asking 'Why me?' I played with the cards I was dealt, the same as everyone else.

'You talk about loneliness, about having a lack of self-confidence, about being, well, depressed, in a lot of ways,' Gina commented. 'In psychology we often think of depression as anger turned inwards.'

'But you don't think I'm clinically depressed,' I said, echoing what she had told me a session or two earlier.

'No,' she admitted, 'I don't think you're clinically depressed. You're just . . . sad.'

'Maybe not forever,' I said. 'Maybe not forever. I have Aisling in my life now, so . . . Besides, if depression is anger turned inwards — I think my family would dispute that I turn my anger inwards!' I laughed a little.

Gina raised her eyebrows. 'I can't imagine you losing the head,' she remarked.

I laughed again. 'Oh, no, I frequently lose the head when I'm at home. I'll have stupid arguments with my parents or sisters. But the thing is — I can't remember a time when I've actually needed to argue over something. I just do it because it feels so good to be able to get angry about anything. Home is the only place where I can do that, though. You go out angry into the world, and you don't keep many friends.

'But I'm trying not to get angry, even at home, anymore,' I concluded. 'My parents and sisters don't deserve it.'

We stayed silent for a few seconds.

Then: 'What was the worst time with your illness?' Gina asked.

I didn't even have to think about that one. 'The final month of my transplant,' I answered, 'the psychosis.'

Gina nodded. 'What was that like for you?'

I described my hallucinations, the fear that had possessed me. 'But it's mostly a blur now,' I added. 'You probably know what I was actually like better than I do.'

'You were . . .' my psychologist hesitated, 'not at all your usual self. The determination in your eyes was gone and there was just this frantic, absolute terror.'

Gina told me that my psychotic episode would have been akin to being on a three-week-long cocaine 'nightmare'.

'How do you feel about that period now?' my therapist prodded.

'I don't know,' I replied. 'Like I said, I don't remember it all. When I think about it, though, I'm still frightened of how easy it is to lose your grip on . . . everything, really.'

Sometimes I think I would like to wake up one morning and have completely forgotten all that I've been through. I suppose each of us feels like that on occasion. A friend once wrote to me that I'd lived through an entire lifetime in two decades. 'You've suffered illness and indignity, loved deeply and heartbreakingly, and almost died', he wrote. And it was true, in a sense, I guess. I hope this doesn't sound arrogant, but, at the age of eighteen, I found myself wondering if there was any emotion, or even any intensity of emotion, left for me to know.

Sometimes, I did feel like a very old man.

Epilogue: 'So'

'What'll you have?' I asked Hugh, one of my closest friends since Bray School Project days. It was the last Friday before Christmas 2003, and the two of us were about to enter a pub. On the road beneath us, shards of broken bottles glinted, and made it seem as though we were standing between two skies: between the stars above, and the stars of glass that were scattered on the tarmac.

We went inside, and ordered pints.

Hugh took a box of cigarettes from his jacket pocket. 'So,' he said, plucking one from the packet, 'you're going to write your story?'

'Yeah,' I replied.

'Well,' Hugh lit his cigarette and took a drag, 'it's not over yet.'

I grinned. 'No.'

Our drinks arrived, and Hugh gestured towards a table by one of the pub's windows. We sauntered over and sat down.

'My story.' I'd spent so much of my life not wanting to be myself. From the young kid wishing he were one of Captain Planet's Planeteers, or wishing he were a superhero who lived inside the Sugarloaf – to the slightly older kid, who still wanted to be Superman. Or, at least, someone with a stronger body.

But this was me. And the truth was, I had discovered a certain strength in the things I'd come through. I gazed out the window beside me, into the blackness of a cold night. For the first time in a long time, I felt like my life was just beginning.

I looked up at Hugh and smiled.

'So,' I began, 'how're you?'